HOW TO FALL IN LOVE WITH YOGA

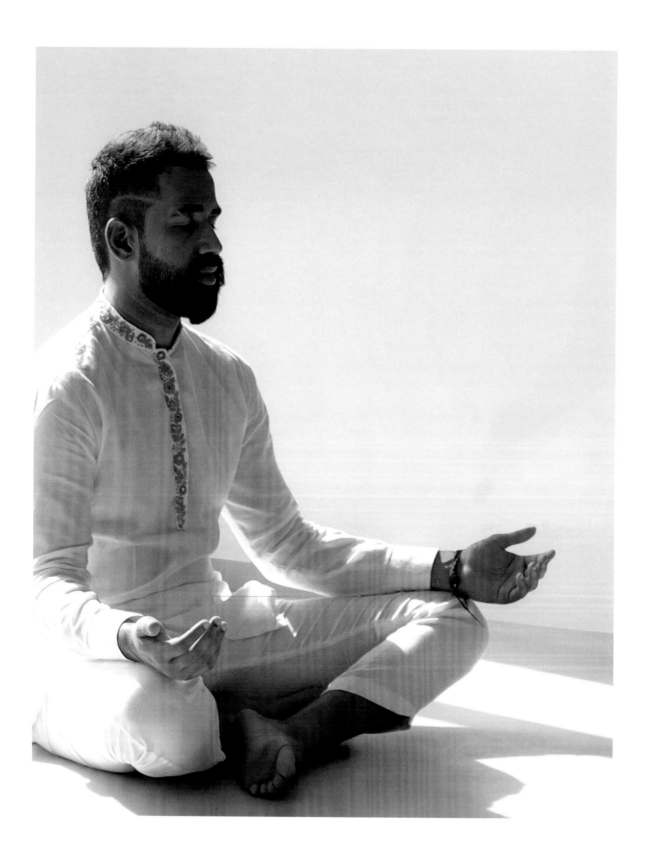

HOW TO FALL IN LOVE WITH YOGA

MOVE BREATHE CONNECT

SARVESH SHASHI

FOREWORD BY MALAIKA ARORA

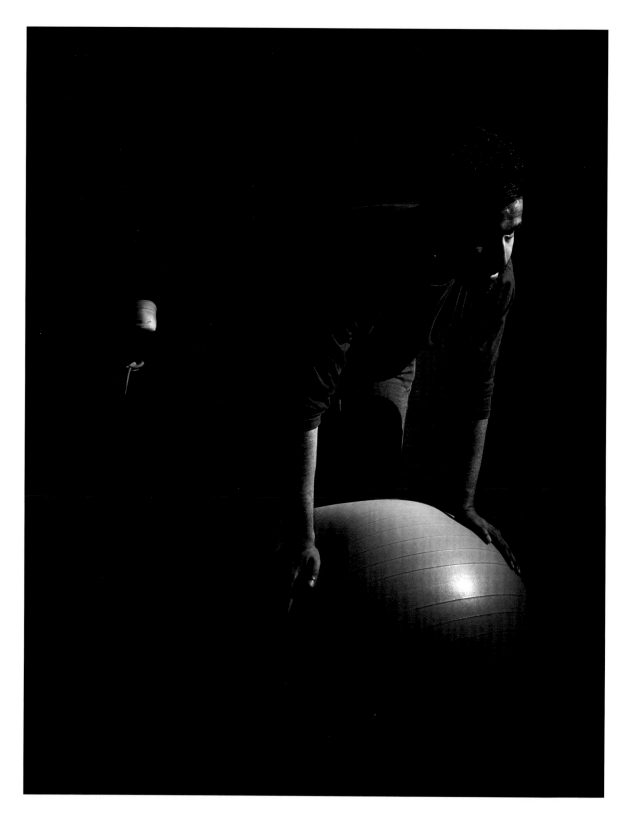

CONTENTS

PUBLISHER'S NOTE:
The ideas, procedures, and suggestions contained in this book are not intended as a substitute for consulting with a qualified medical practitioner. Always consult your doctor before starting a fitness regime if you have any health concerns. Neither the author nor the publisher shall be liable or responsible for any loss or damage allegedly arising from any information or suggestion in this book.

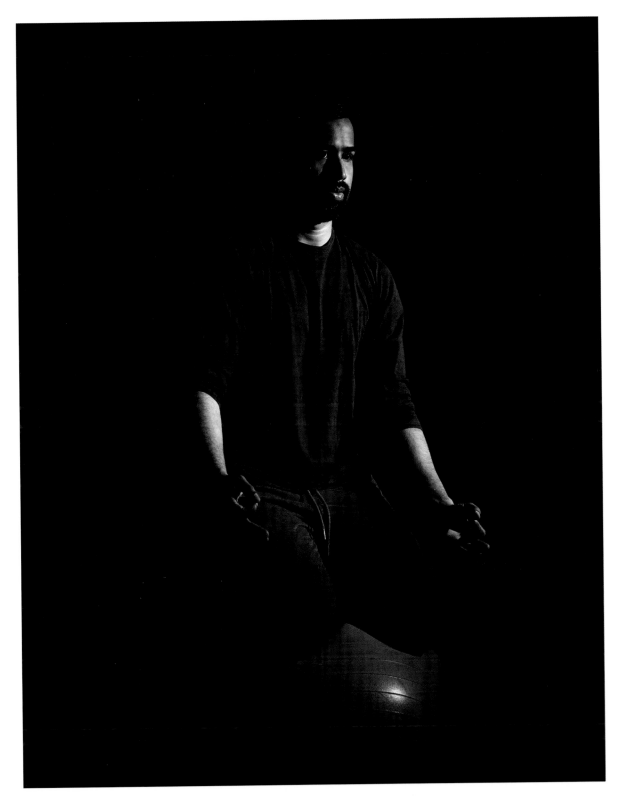

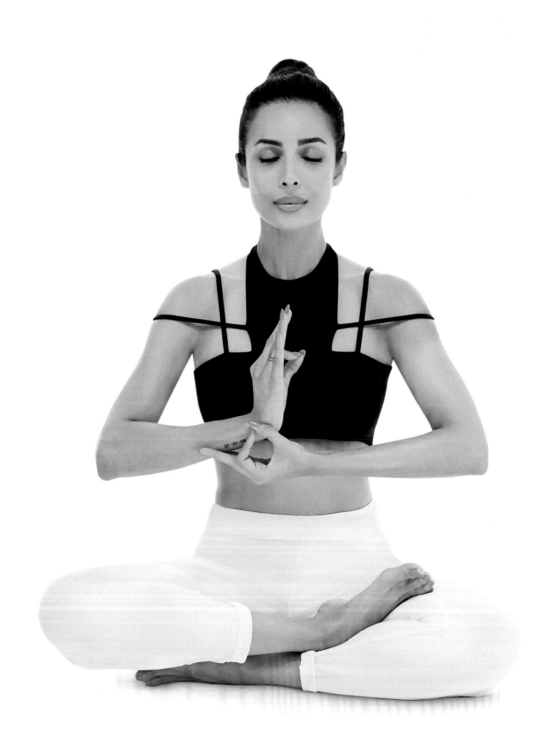

FOREWORD

Sarvesh, I have known you for many years now. Apart from being my business partner, you are also like my younger brother, my best friend, and my constant yoga partner. I feel immense joy and pride as I pen down a few heartfelt words as a foreword to your book, *How to Fall in Love with Yoga*. As I read through the amazing synopsis of your work, I couldn't help but feel excited for what lies ahead for all those fortunate enough to discover its pages.

Your book promises to be a profound and transformative journey into the world of yoga. What truly resonates with me is your unwavering dedication to making yoga accessible to everyone regardless of their experience level. In a world often clouded with complexity, your holistic and inclusive approach to yoga is a breath of fresh air.

As someone who has closely witnessed your yoga journey, I know first-hand the authenticity and passion you bring to this ancient practice. Your personal experiences in the book are a testament to your deep connection with yoga, making it not just about the body, but also a journey of the mind and the soul.

Your carefully written book, designed to resonate with readers and guide them on their own path of self-discovery and well-being, is both thoughtful and inspiring. Your dedication to address mental health, weight management, overall fitness, and women's health through the wisdom of yoga is highly commendable. The exploration of meditative practices that nurture inner peace is much needed in our fast-paced world.

I am particularly looking forward to your practical guide for executing asanas at home. Your book is bound to motivate numerous individuals to begin their exploration towards wellness. Your commitment to staying true to the authentic and original forms of yoga, while infusing it with a youthful and accessible flavour, is a great way to reach out to a broader audience.

Along with this book, you have also crafted a roadmap to a healthier, happier, and more balanced life. I have no doubt that your words will inspire a lot of people to embark on their own transformative yoga journeys.

Congratulations on this incredible endeavour!

MALAIKA ARORA
Co-founder of Diva Yoga and actor

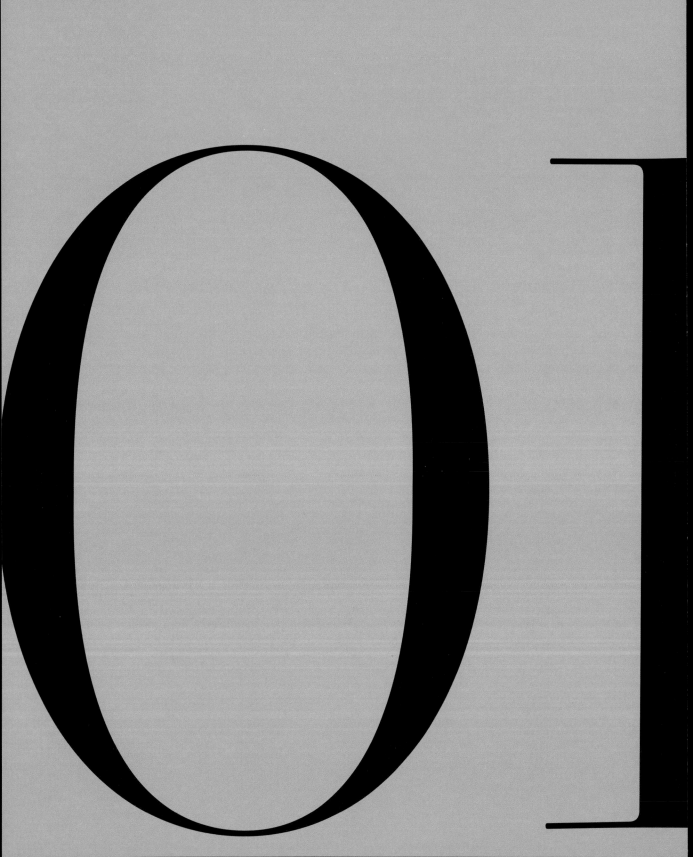

"

Yoga is like music: the rhythm of the body,
the melody of the mind, and the harmony
of the soul create the symphony of life.

B.K.S. IYENGAR, FOUNDER OF IYENGAR YOGA

"

YOGA: **A WAY OF LIFE**

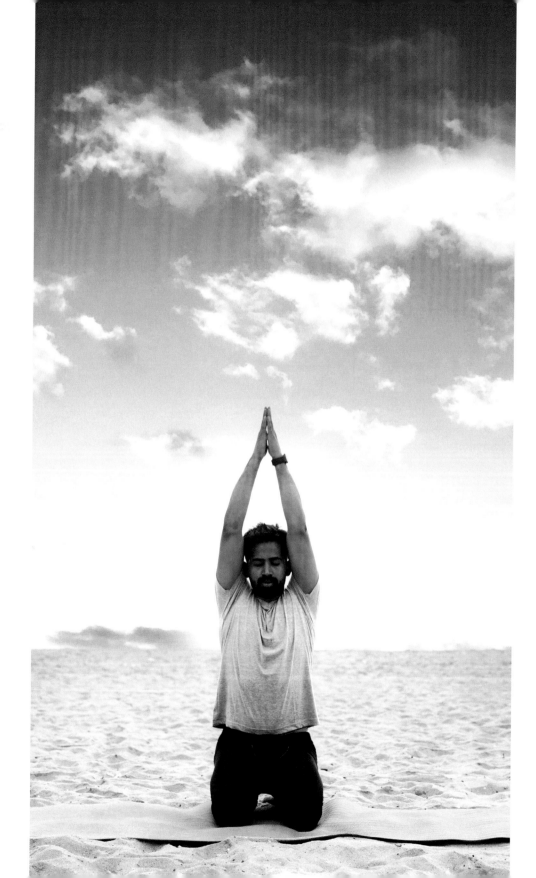

BECOMING A YOGI

I was 17 when I met Vijayendra, the man who would become my guru – the dispeller of darkness. I had just joined a yoga class with my father, and there he was, this man, clad in saffron clothes, with a flowing beard and long hair. He reminded me of a godman, those that claim to enlighten the masses and profess divine powers. But, as I interacted with him, I realized that though there was no halo or third eye to behold, he had immense knowledge to impart. I didn't know it then, but he would change my life. I think this was when I started falling in love with yoga.

My guru taught me that yoga was more than a series of movements, that pranayama, or breathing techniques, ground you, and that the true meaning of *dhyana*, or meditation, was not to sit in silence and let your thoughts run amok, but to bring yourself to the present, let go of negativity, and become a vessel, almost, for peace and joy to seep in.

This wasn't my first brush with yoga. I first learnt yoga when I was 6. It was used as bait – I dreamt of playing cricket for India and bringing home the World Cup, and yoga, my parents told me, would help me become a better sportsperson. I decided to try it, but, really, I was going through the motions. It was a means to an end.

When I look back now, I think of my life as a journey in two parts. The first were the years before I turned 17, marked by the four As – arrogance, anger, attitude, and anxiety. Then there were the years after I met my guru. It was only while taking his class that I realized that yoga could have a deeper meaning and hold much more space in my life.

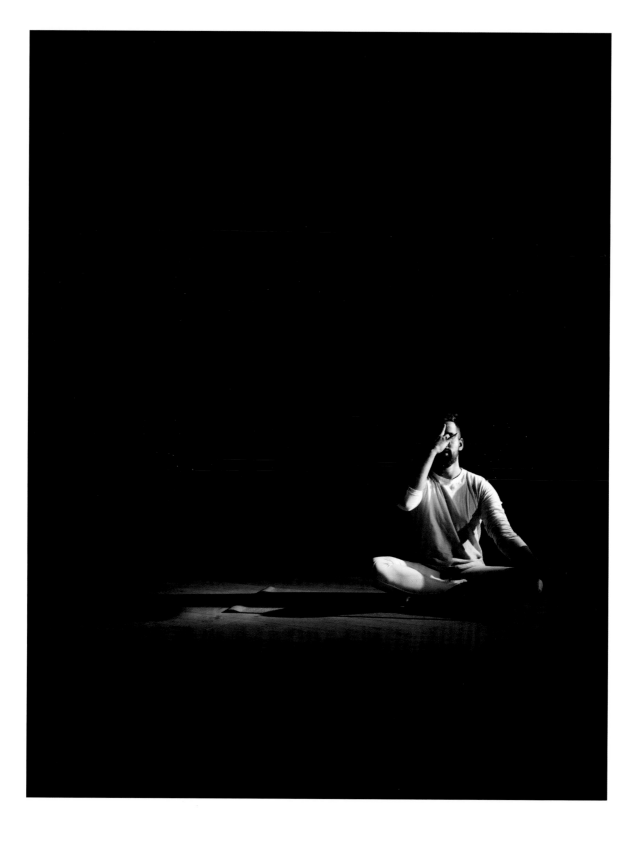

> "
> With every fall, there is a rise.
> With every change, there is growth.
> With every hurt, there is hope.
> With every ending, there is a new beginning.
> "

I was young and finding my place in the world, and the practice of yoga helped me become familiar with the rhythms of my mind, body, and the world. This came from committing to the practice, from allowing the discipline of yoga to become a part of me. It did not come easily, of course.

I began by setting small goals, sticking to a sadhana, or disciplined practice, such as doing a flow regularly for three days, then seven, then harder sadhanas such as being silent for 10 days. I threw myself into yoga and worked my way up to 40 days. By 18, I had undertaken five disciplined practices. These were no intoxication, non-violence, no mental or physical stealing, no lies (not even white lies), and celibacy. I've done sadhanas such as the candle *trataka*, the mirror *trataka*, *chakra trataka*, going without any form of electronics or human touch for days at a time, and meditating for six to nine hours a day. I realized that yoga was no longer a means to an end, but a spiritual endeavour. It had become a way of life. This shift in perspective was transformational and I learnt to love myself.

One can only feel and express love for creatures and the environment if one knows how to love oneself. Yoga brings conscious awareness: a deeper understanding of the way one breathes while experiencing the states of mind, to be able to feel the shift in one's energy while encountering various situations.

It doesn't matter who you are, what you weigh, how old you are, or where you come from, yoga embraces everyone. It is like that quote which states that yoga is not a journey "on" the mat, but "of" the mat – it is a path into oneself, it is enlightenment.

After all, there is a yogi in all of us.

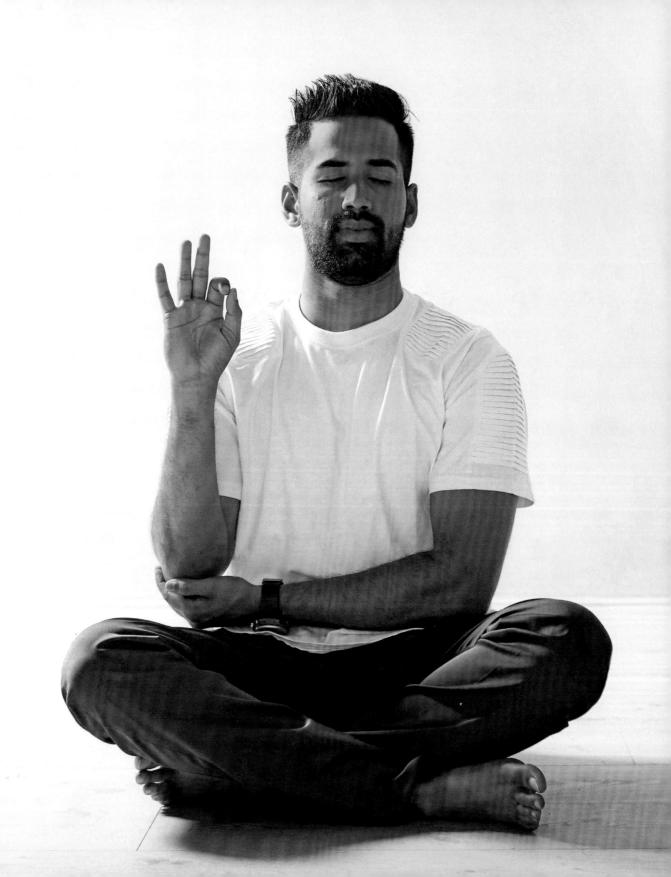

THE PATH TOWARDS WELLNESS

Yoga is many things. It is pranayama (breathwork), *dhyana* (meditation), and asana (exercises in the form of postures), but it is also intention, discipline, and commitment. At its root, yoga is "union" or the "union of dualities", as the *Yogabija*, a seminal work on Hatha yoga that traces its origins to the 1st century CE, calls it. Simply, it is the union of the mind, body, and soul.

Any activity that encourages one to be present and connected with the present, with each other, and with themselves is a part of this union. I see yoga as a way of life. It is as important as brushing one's teeth or eating breakfast every day.

Often the practice of yoga can lead one towards rigidity of the type of form, but I think the word itself tells one to be fluid. There are no bounds to yoga, to impose some would be a disservice to its powers. Yoga helps one to love and be kind to oneself, and in turn disseminates this love and kindness to others in the world.

YOU ARE THE IDEAL

Yoga is simply a matter of finding your fit and approaching it with the right intention. It is a way into knowing and loving oneself – one's body and mind. As with any outward physical or mental interaction, there are certain contraindications to the practice as well. I would not suggest doing certain asanas in case of injuries, for example. But, this is where the limitation ends.

Intentions encompass many possibilities. Choose to cultivate focus on breath, think about what you are grateful for, or repeat a specific affirmation or mantra. Setting an intention before starting is a foundational and an incredible tool to prepare oneself for a new goal, or fresh mind space.

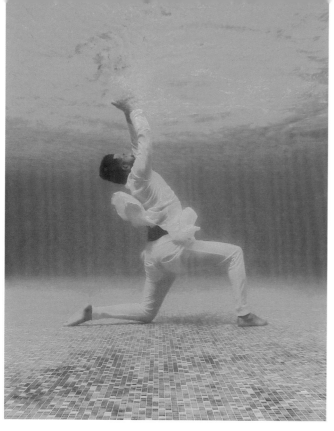
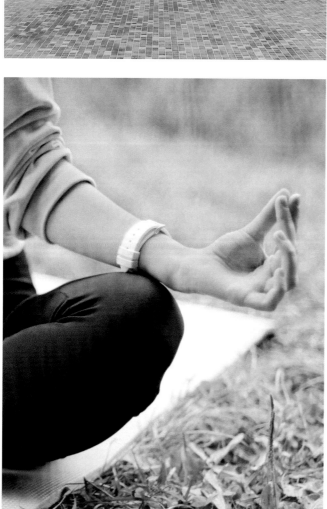
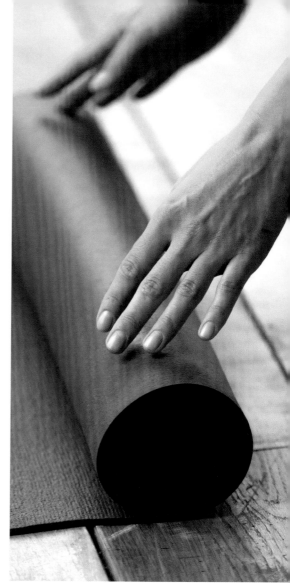
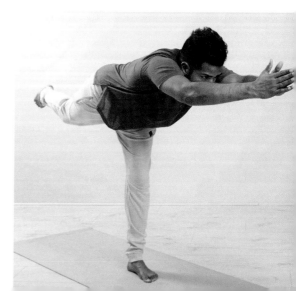

Allow yourself the space to embrace the practice in its entirety. We can all do this, no matter who we are or where we are starting.

A client once told me how grateful they were to have found yoga, because they felt the safest and the most comfortable when cocooned in its practice. Stories like that are why I love yoga so much. It has been fulfilling to watch people fall in love with this way of life, and it gives me joy to see how much yoga has benefited them.

If there was one piece of advice I could give, it would be to imbibe this: there is no ideal frame of mind, ideal body, or ideal person who can set out on this path. Understand your starting point, set an intention, and see the magic unfold.

SETTING GOALS WITH YOGA

The best part of yoga is that its goals can be flexible. A rigid goal is deciding to tone the muscles in one's arms in, say, 30 days. But it is the flexible goals such as the decision to improve one's health that provides the space to make and sustain effective change over a period of time. It takes discipline and commitment. Anything that hinders the journey to a goal, whether an external substance or an action, needs to be understood and set aside.

Some believe that the definition of success should change from owning material goods to simply waking up in the morning with a smile on your face. This is a perfect, flexible goal to begin with. Equally valid are goals that help one lose weight, improve mental health, or target fitness at large. Ultimately, it is one's best effort that counts. Intensity of practice will only fuel the mind and body until a point, but to commit to one's goals and to yoga for life, one needs regularity. I have, for long, believed that 20 minutes of practice every day will go a longer way than 2 hours for only a week.

RESET, REJUVENATE, AND REFRESH

Yoga has the most impact on cleaning the nervous system and the gut. Between these lie a multitude of ambitions. Goals can cover different facets of one's health and wellness, but there are four that draw people to yoga the most: mental health, weight loss, women's health, and general fitness.

For as long as there has been society, and human life, there has been stress. Negative emotions – the unrest of everyday life, the agonizing over the future – have always affected us. Yoga, however, helps one move away from all of this. It anchors one to the present. It centres the mind and body and creates dissonance from the turmoil. Balance is key, and yoga is all about that.

Through pranayama, *dhyana*, and asanas, one can naturally ease stress and even actively feel the knots in our muscles, or the tension leaving the body. Yoga pulls focus inwards. It fosters self-reflection and a heightened awareness of oneself. This allows one the space to tackle one's emotions and embrace the necessary change, often transforming the way one views the world. The journey towards fitness and weight loss is an ongoing one. It is a combination of many different things – from eating nourishing food, doing the right exercises, and finding time for rest and recovery, to practising self-care and building self-confidence. Yoga asanas burn calories, aid in digestion, regulate metabolism, and target stubborn areas of the body, but they also provide the tools to strike the perfect balance between factors such as mental clarity, better sleep, peace with oneself, and rejuvenation, which are necessary to meet fitness goals.

Practising yoga is just as preventative as it can be healing. By focusing on underlying causes, not only can it reduce the severity of many ailments, especially those that affect women, but it can also be a deterrent for certain factors that may cause problems in the future. Painful menstruation, menopause, and hormonal imbalances are ailments that can be eased with regular practice.

When I say that yoga is transformational, or that yoga can help everyone, it is not to claim it is a magic pill. Yoga cannot join a broken bone, as that needs medicine.

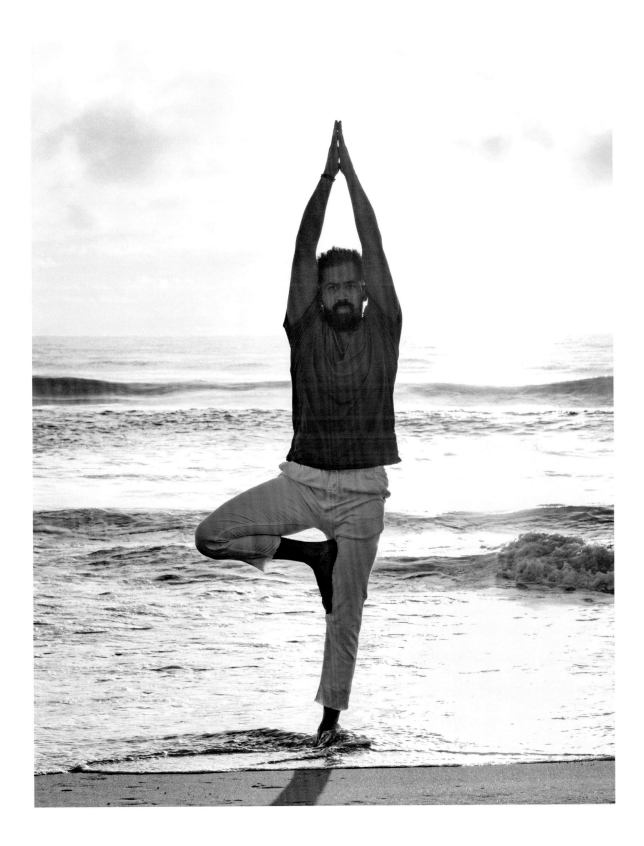

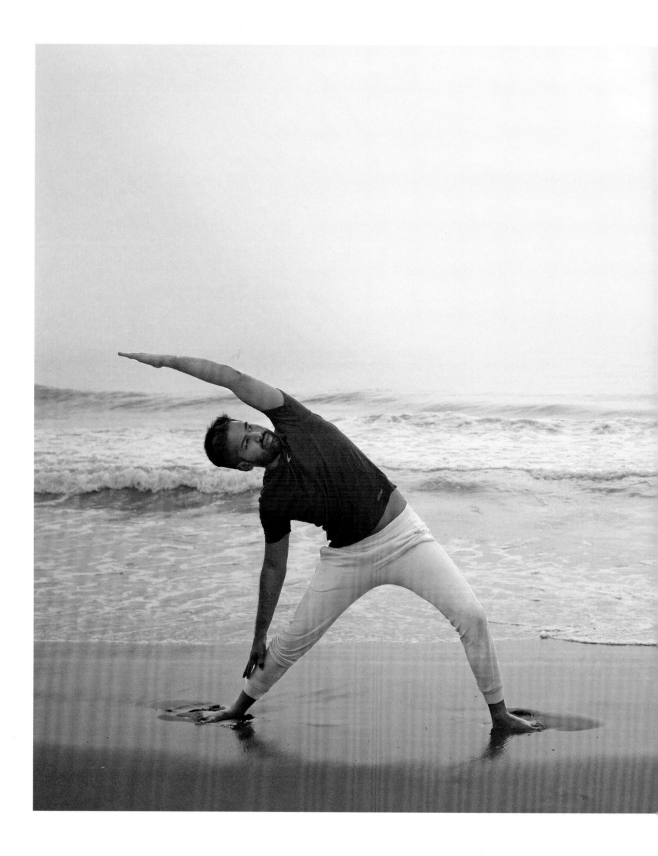

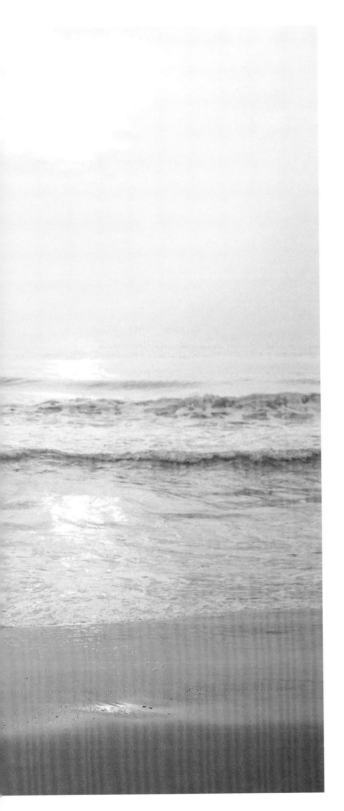

However, yoga can step in after medicine has done its job. It can help with faster healing and restore motion to injured limbs.

MEASURING CHANGE

Once one embraces the wholesome, holistic nature of yoga, the limitlessness of the mind and body begins to reveal itself. So how does one count this or monitor the intentions to see if they are bearing fruit? The only way is through evolution and change. This does not need to be something big. Celebrating the alleviation of chronic pain is impactful, but so is something as simple as being able to go to bed five minutes earlier than usual. I always say, a week after you start practising yoga regularly, think back to how many times you woke up feeling more fulfilled and less anxious about the day, or just found yourself breathing in a more relaxed manner through the day.

Count the small wins, and then commit to another week. Before you know it, you will be well into your journey of wellness.

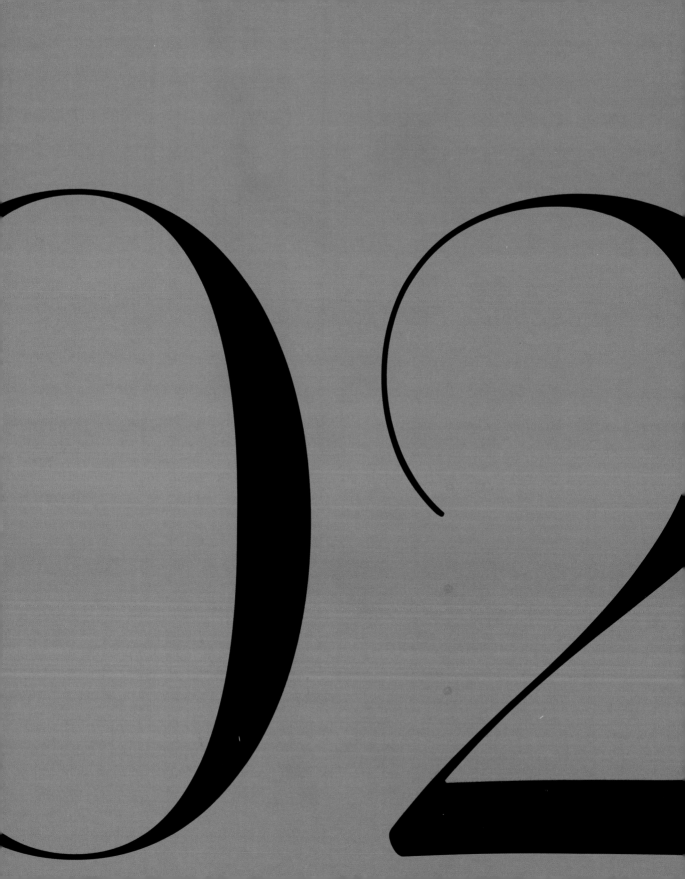

"
Undisturbed calmness of mind is attained
by cultivating friendliness toward the happy,
compassion for the unhappy, delight in the virtuous,
and indifference toward the wicked.

PATANJALI, AUTHOR, MYSTIC, AND PHILOSOPHER, c.401–500 CE

"

UNWIND

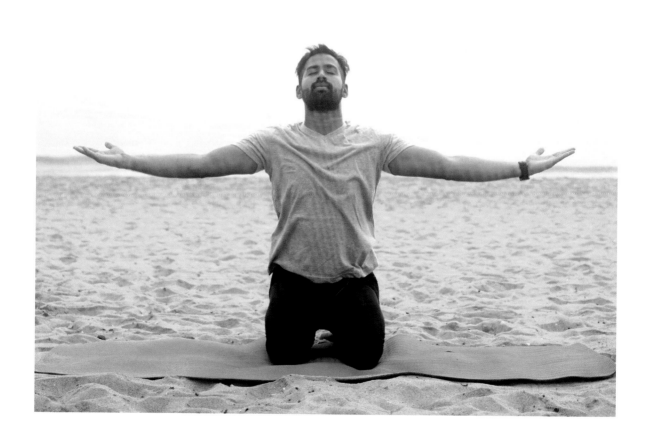

MENTAL HEALTH THROUGH YOGA

Each individual's path is unique, but through yoga, everyone can find the strength to heal, grow, and flourish. In a world that often demands perfection, the best thing one can do is remember that it is okay not to be okay all the time. Yogic belief postulates that every practice, like life itself, is made up of highs and lows. It is okay to stumble; what matters is one's willingness to rise again.

Mental health is an intrinsic part of wellness, and as one sets out on this journey, yoga can become one's sanctuary, offering solace and support in times of need. Much of the struggles we face when it comes to our mental health stem from uncertainty and anxiety about the future, and worrying about what has already passed. Through *dhyana* (meditation) and pranayama (breathwork), uncover

the calming influence of yoga on racing thoughts and anxiety. Through stretching asanas and exercise flows, one can release pent-up emotions and heal emotional wounds. There are many different types of meditation and breathwork exercises, such as gratefulness meditation, the *Trataka* with a candle (see p71), *Dirga Pranayama* (see pp68–69), and more, some of which have been illustrated in the book. Their aim is to heighten our ability to focus and concentrate. This removes distractions from the path and aids in grounding us and promoting mindfulness.

When engaging with regular yogic practice, one must try to embrace vulnerabilities and be gentle with the self so as to replace self-criticism with self-love. Regular practice does not necessarily translate to practicing yoga with intensity, but refers to cultivating and perfecting the basics which are the building blocks of more advanced practice, should one wish to attempt it.

My journey is replete with examples of yoga keeping me present, grounded, and thriving. It is only through this practice that I have found my feet, time and time again. In 2020, as the COVID-19 pandemic set in, my work took a hit as it did for many people around the world. I felt out of balance watching the unwanted changes take over. I did not know what to do or what the future held for me. Yoga kept me calm. It brought balance and taught me that as long as there was breath in my body, things would be all right.

Achieving one's mental health goal with yoga is possible. Asanas such as *Savasana* (see pp66-67) are the best starting point to clear the mind and see the stress dissipate. *Anulom Vilom* (see p109) is a great pranayama for regulating breath and *Bitilasana* (see p128) helps to relieve stored tension in the back muscles. Another great asana for calming racing thoughts is the *Anand Balasana* (see p156) or the child's pose.

There are simple ways to facilitate this journey and make it an even better experience for the self, such as practicing outdoors. Fresh air and nature are great motivators. Adding music and musical relaxation at the end of a session can also be a good way to calm the mind. Tailor routines for mental health by including at least one pranayama and *dhyana* flow. In fact, I suggest ending all flows with *Dhyana* (see pp72-73) to enable a smooth transition from yoga to one's daily routine.

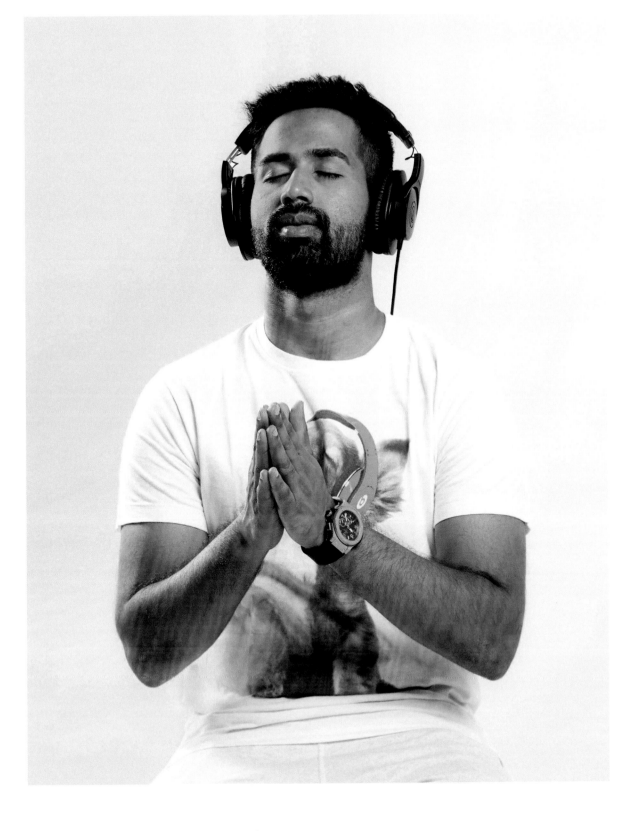

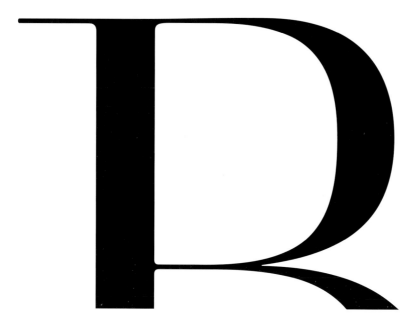

BREATHE for five minutes every day. Understand the rhythm of your breath and employ the right techniques – expand your chest as you inhale and contract it as you exhale. Be measured and deliberate for a few minutes as you experience breathwork through *Anulom Vilom*, or "alternate nostril breathing". Allow yourself to be engulfed in the meditative power of focused breathing as it brings peace, calm, and heightened awareness to you. Deep breaths serve as anchors to ground you in the present, so breathe with the right yogic technique for a week and you will experience the difference yourself.

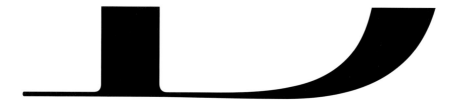

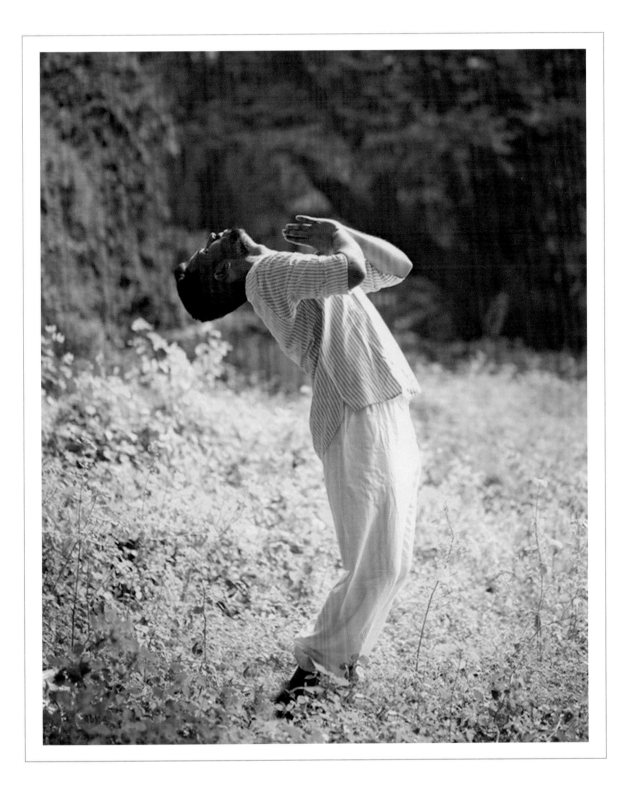

UNWIND FLOW

Yoga is a restorative tool for fostering a sense of calm and relaxation. This sequence gently guides from *Sukhasana* (see pp34–35) to *Dhyana* (see pp72–73), and helps reduce stress and anxiety, and bring relaxation. Dedicated practice of this flow will also help one improve sleep, enhance concentration, and boost cognitive function.

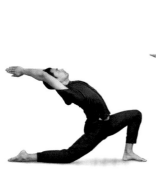

5 **Anjaneyasana**
Pages 42–43

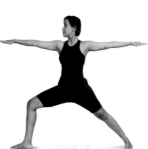

6 **Virabhadrasana II**
Pages 46–47

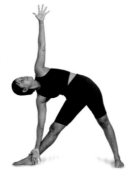

7 **Trikonasana**
Pages 48–49

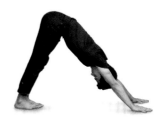

8 **Adho Mukha Shvanasana** *Pages 52–53*

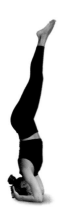

13 **Adha Sirsasana**
Pages 60–61

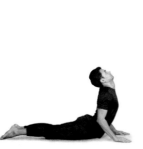

14 **Bhujangasana**
Pages 62–63

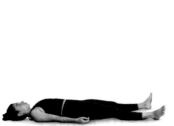

15 **Savasana**
Pages 66–67

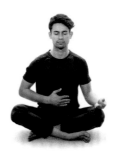

16 **Dirga Pranayama**
Pages 68–69

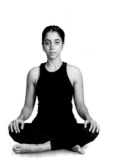

1 Sukhasana
Pages 34–35

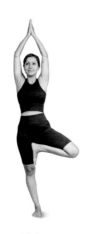

2 Vriksasana
Pages 36–37

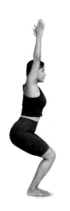

3 Utkatasana
Pages 38–39

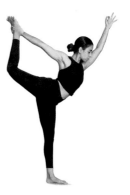

4 Natarajasana
Pages 40–41

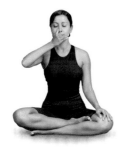

9 Bakasana
Pages 54–55

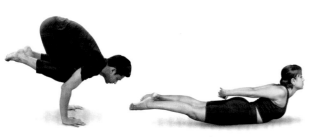

10 Salabhasana
Page 56

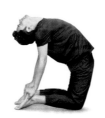

11 Ustrasana
Page 57

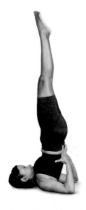

12 Sarvangasana
Pages 58–59

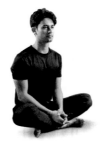

17 Single Nostril Breathing
Page 70

18 Trataka
Page 71

End every yoga flow, or routine, with a few moments of meditation. This will bring the mind and body back to a regulated sense of calm and foster equilibrium. Dedicated practice brings an understanding of the self and fosters steadiness of the mind and body.

19 Dhyana
Pages 72–73

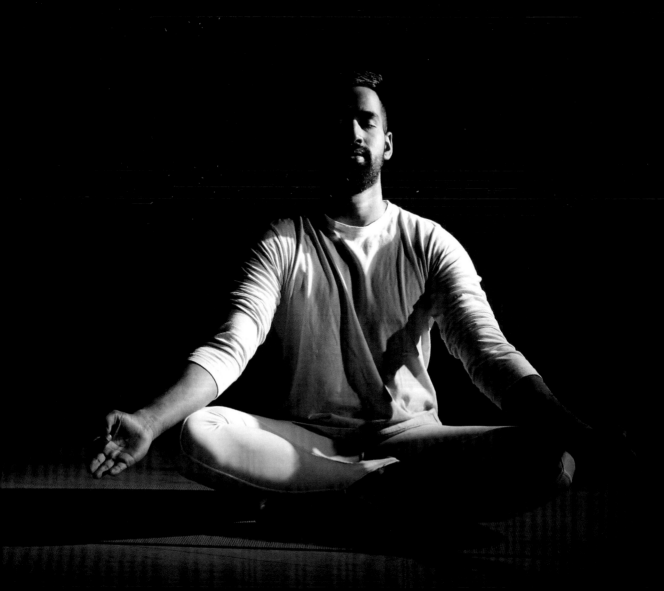

> "
> Breathe deeply, relax, and
> release any doubts and fears
> to your higher self, and find
> the peace within.
> "

SUKHASANA

The cross-legged, seated posture, also known as the "easy sitting pose", or *Sukhasana*, is the foundation for several asanas. It is considered one of the most basic poses in yoga and meditation.

BENEFITS & CARE

Sukhasana aids in focused breathing. It also eases lower back and knee pain. Avoid this asana in case of previous knee or hip injuries or chronic joint pain.

IN FOCUS

Sukhasana is one of the best poses for meditation and has a great positive impact on mental health. It has a relaxing effect on the mind and body, improves focus and concentration, and reduces anxiety.

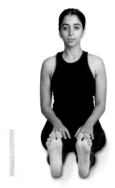

Sit with both legs stretched out in front. The neck and back should remain straight at all times.

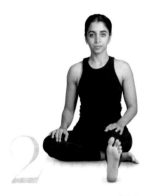

Keep the spine straight, fold one leg at the knee, and bring the sole of the foot to rest under the other thigh.

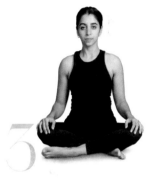

Repeat the same movement with the other leg and adjust the seating position so as to feel minimal pressure on both ankles.

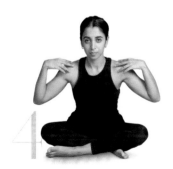

Place the palms on the shoulders and gently move the shoulder blades back and down. The head should be raised with the crown facing up.

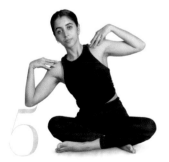

Move the body back and forth and side to side a few times to ensure that the shoulders are squarely above the hips. Breathe normally while moving.

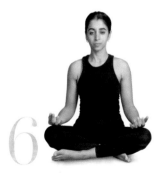

To rest, bring the palms to the knees. Repeat the movement as many times as needed to feel "loose" enough to begin the other asanas.

THE AIM OF YOGA IS TO CALM THE CHAOS OF CONFLICTING IMPULSES.

B.K.S. IYENGAR, FOUNDER OF IYENGAR YOGA

VRIKSASANA

The "tree pose", or *Vriksasana*, derives its name from the final, graceful tree-like posture. A basic balancing yoga pose, it is taught to beginners and practised by expert practitioners. It emphasizes the strengthening of the body's core.

BENEFITS & CARE

Vriksasana aids in maintaining balance, equilibrium, good posture, and concentration. Do not practise in case of high blood pressure, migraine, arthritis, or a history of hip surgery.

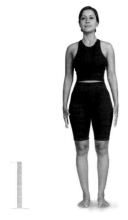

1 Stand straight and plant both feet firmly on the ground. Feel the even distribution of weight over the four corners of each foot.

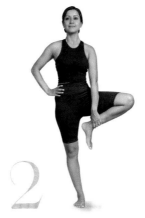

2 Shifting weight on the right foot, raise the left foot off the ground (hold with a hand if needed). Keep the right leg straight but don't lock the right knee.

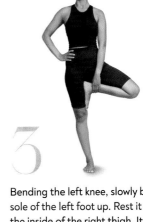

3 Bending the left knee, slowly bring the sole of the left foot up. Rest it along the inside of the right thigh. It can also rest below the knee but never beside it.

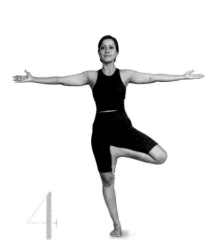

4 Apply pressure with the thigh to the foot and vice versa. Fix gaze at an object at eye level, while keeping hips stable and body straight. Raise the arms to the side.

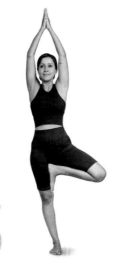

5 Gently raise the arms above the head and bring the palms together. This is the final pose. Hold for at least five deep breaths, then slowly relax.

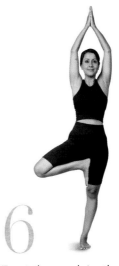

6 To exit the pose, bring the raised leg to the ground. Redistribute body weight, and slowly repeat the asana on the opposite side.

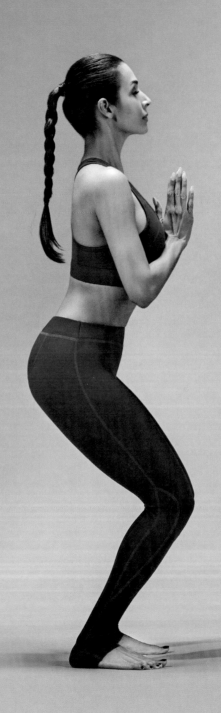

UTKATASANA

This standing pose is also called the "powerful pose" or the "fierce seat pose" and has an impact on the lower body, especially the spine, thighs, calves, and ankles. *Utkatasana* is also good for postural awareness and balance. In the final position, the body resembles a bolt of lightning.

BENEFITS & CARE

Utkatasana activates the core and works on muscles in the lower back, thighs, and calves. It aids in digestion and promotes wellbeing. Contraindications include high or low blood pressure, respiratory complications, chronic lower back or knee pain, and ligament injuries. It should also be avoided if menstruating.

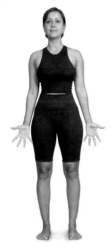

1 Take a standing position. Plant both feet firmly on the ground and distribute weight equally on both soles of the feet to stay balanced.

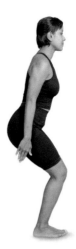

2 Turn towards the shorter edge of the mat. Keep the feet shoulder-width apart and push the hips back so they protrude slightly. Bend the knees as though sitting on a chair.

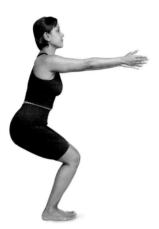

3 Squat as low as possible while keeping feet parallel. Raise both hands up to the shoulder level and extend straight to bring balance.

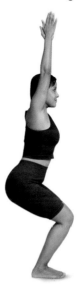

4 Slowly raise hands over the head. The neck and spine should be straight in this final pose. Hold it for five deep breaths, then relax.

NATARAJASANA

The "lord of dance pose" is named after Nataraja, Hindu god Shiva's form as the divine cosmic dancer. The asana is great for back-bending and balancing. Advanced practitioners perform a more complicated version, where, in the ultimate pose, the sole of the raised foot comes close to the crown of the head. It has been modified here to suit all levels of practitioners.

BENEFITS & CARE

Great for muscles in the legs, hips, and core, *Natarajasana* also helps the mind to focus. Those with back pain, heart issues, high blood pressure, vertigo, ulcers, colitis, or hernia should avoid it.

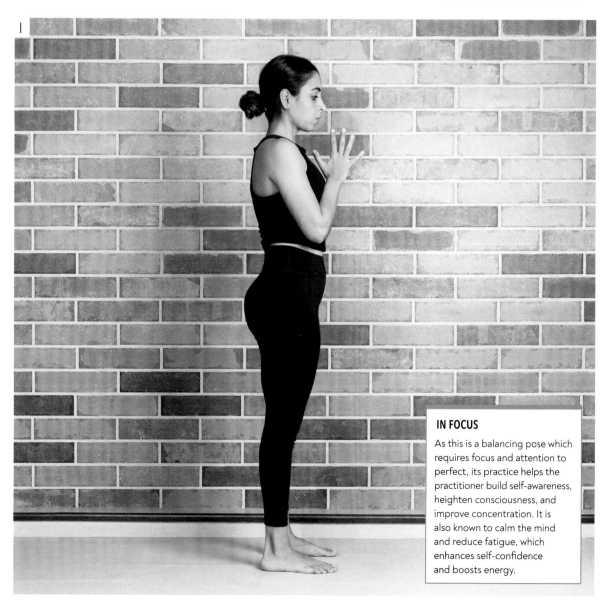

1

IN FOCUS

As this is a balancing pose which requires focus and attention to perfect, its practice helps the practitioner build self-awareness, heighten consciousness, and improve concentration. It is also known to calm the mind and reduce fatigue, which enhances self-confidence and boosts energy.

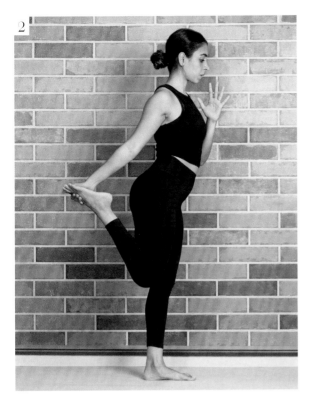

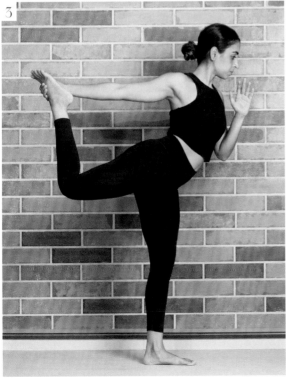

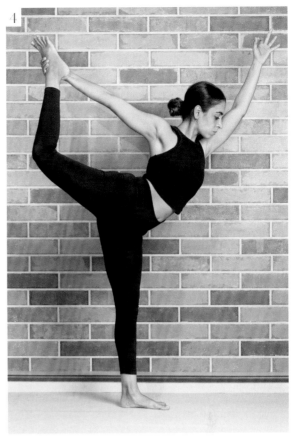

1 Stand facing the shorter edge of the mat. Take a deep breath. Join the palms and keep eyes fixed on a single object. Get ready to balance on one leg.

2 Bend the right leg and bring it close to the glutes while holding the foot with the right palm. Carefully move the left hand freely while maintaining balance. The gaze should remain fixed.

3 Concentrate all the body weight on the left leg. Slowly extend the right leg as far back as possible.

4 Raise the right leg higher, while also raising the left hand. Raise them as high as possible. Hold this pose for five breaths. Return to the starting position and repeat with the left leg.

ANJANEYASANA

Translating to "son of Anjani", a reference to Hanumana, the monkey-god, this asana is also called the "low lunge pose" due to it being a lunging back-bending posture. The practice of *Anjaneyasana* stretches muscles in the groin, hamstrings, and the front and back of both legs. A variation of this popular and versatile asana is also sometimes included in the *Surya Namaskar* (see pp182–185).

BENEFITS & CARE

Great for core muscles, hamstrings, quadriceps, and the hip, *Anjaneyasana* improves flexibility and relieves tension and stress from the body. Those with neck or back problems, high blood pressure, or hip, knee, or groin injuries should avoid it.

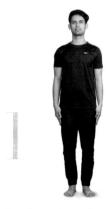

Stand straight on the mat with feet shoulder-width apart. The arms should be relaxed on either side of the body.

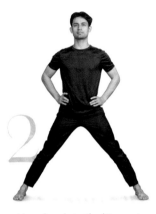

Move hands to the hips and spread both legs as much as is possible without discomfort.

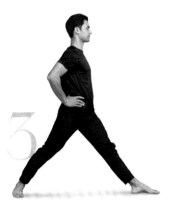

Turn the torso to the left. Rotate the left foot outwards by 90 degrees. Take the time to find balance in this posture.

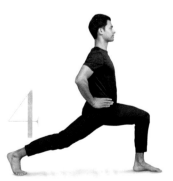

Bend the left knee and raise the right heel off the ground. It should be easier to balance in this position.

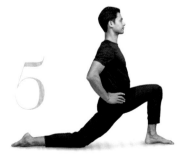

On an exhale, lower the right knee to the ground. The toes should point backwards.

> "
> In *Anjaneyasana*, you curve the body into
> the shape of a crescent moon – often called
> the symbol of yoga.
>
> LUCY LIDELL, NARAYANI RABINOVITCH AND GIRIS RABINOVITCH,
> *THE BOOK OF YOGA* (1983)
> "

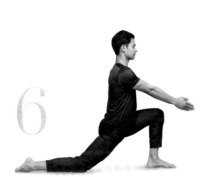

6

On an inhale, join both hands in the
front of the body. Raise them upwards
as if drawing a circle around the body.

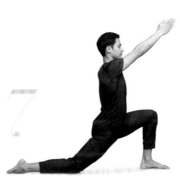

7

While moving the arms in a circle,
begin to lean back. Keep the knee
and feet flat and maintain balance.

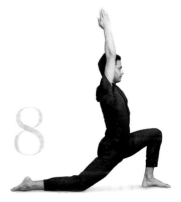

8

Pause when the arms are positioned
straight above the head and take a
deep breath.

9

Bend as far back as possible without pain
in the lower back. Lift the chin high and
keep the eyes skywards. Enjoy the stretch
for five breaths, then bend forwards on
all fours to exit. Repeat on the other side.

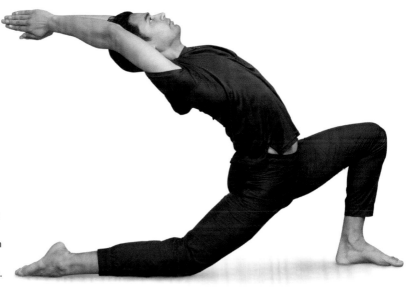

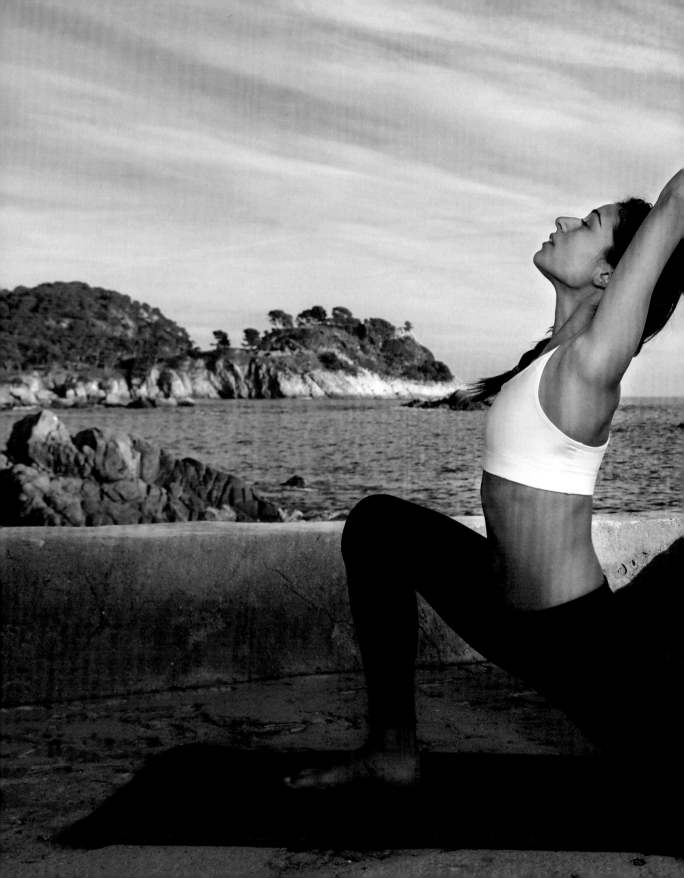

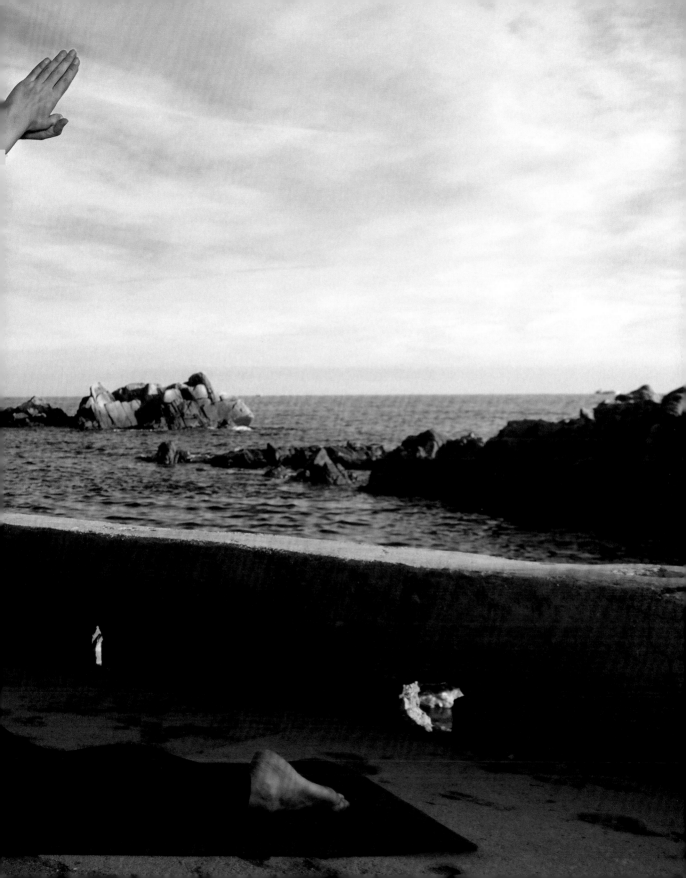

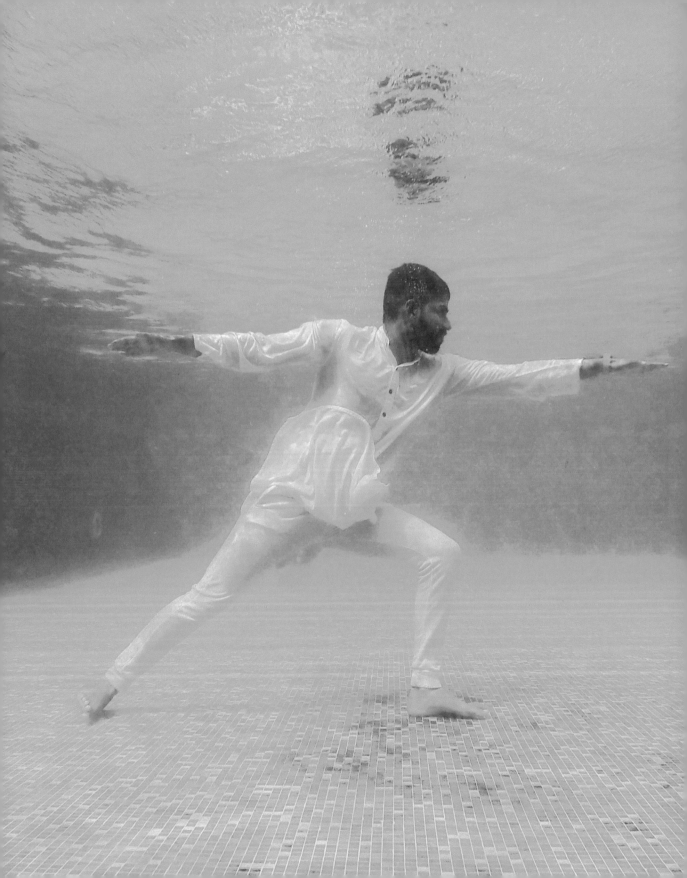

VIRABHADRASANA II

Named after the fierce mythological warrior Virabhadra, a human incarnation of the Hindu god Shiva, this asana is particularly beneficial. The *Virabhadrasana II*, or "warrior II", is a standing yoga posture that strengthens the legs, torso, and spine, and stretches the shoulders, chest, and groin. In this pose, the practitioner's gaze, or *drishti*, must remain calm and steadily upon the hand in front.

BENEFITS & CARE

Impacts quadriceps, thighs, glutes, hips, and shoulders. It improves balance, posture, flexibility, reduces stress, and relieves stored tension. Those with recent or chronic hip, knee, or shoulder injuries should avoid performing the asana.

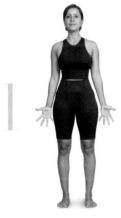

Face the long side of the mat and stand straight. The feet should be parallel to one another. Hands should be on either side of the body.

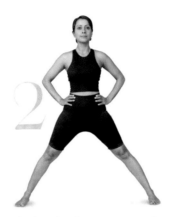

Slowly widen the stance as much as possible without discomfort. Place the hands on the hips.

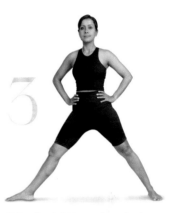

Point the right toe outwards at a 90-degree angle. Slightly turn the torso outwards as well. Keep the gaze fixed in front.

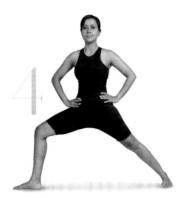

Bend the right knee such that it extends over the right ankle. Equally distribute body weight throughout both legs.

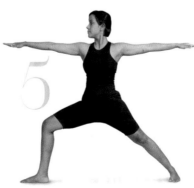

Raise both arms and turn the gaze towards the right hand. Hold the stance for five deep breaths. Release and continue on the opposite side.

IN FOCUS

The work on the physical level in this asana can translate to work on the mental level as well. The intense stretch relieves the tension stored in the muscles and brings a refreshing sense of calm. With regular practice, the body learns to relax and hold its strength throughout different areas of the body.

TRIKONASANA

Trikonasana, or the "triangle pose", is called so because of the triangular shape formed between the hand, hip, and foot, when one achieves the final pose. It has many variations in different traditions of yoga, but all variants focus on side stretches and the improvement of the practitioner's spinal flexibility.

BENEFITS & CARE

Trikonasana strengthens muscles in the legs, hips, back, shoulders, and chest. It reduces stress and increases energy levels. Those with previous neck and back injuries, chronic migraine, or blood pressure issues should take care when performing the asana or avoid it completely.

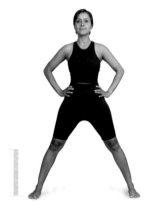

Stand with feet three-feet apart and place hands on the hips. The space between the feet can change based on comfort and one's height.

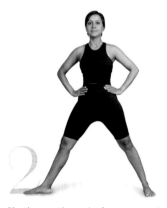

Slowly turn the right foot outwards at a 90-degree angle to the left foot. Maintain the gaze at an object at eye level and stay balanced.

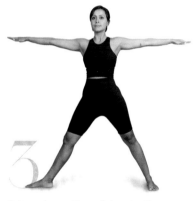

Raise arms until parallel to the floor and in line with each other. Bend to the side and reach for the right ankle with the right hand.

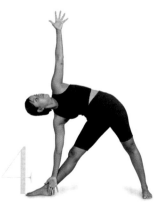

In the final pose, the right hand is on the right ankle, the left hand is raised to the sky, and the gaze is upwards, set upon the left palm.

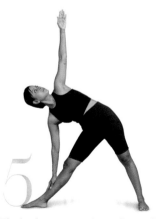

The body must not droop forwards and arms must be taut for an intense stretch on the side. If needed, place hand on the shin. Repeat the same on the other side.

IN FOCUS

Trikonasana fosters energy flow through the body, bringing balance and calmness to the mind. While practising the asana, the practitioner needs to be fully focused and aware of the self, as is exhibited by the steady gaze upwards, focused on the raised palm.

YOGA IS
THE JOURNEY
OF THE SELF,
THROUGH THE SELF,
TO THE SELF.

THE BHAGAVAD GITA

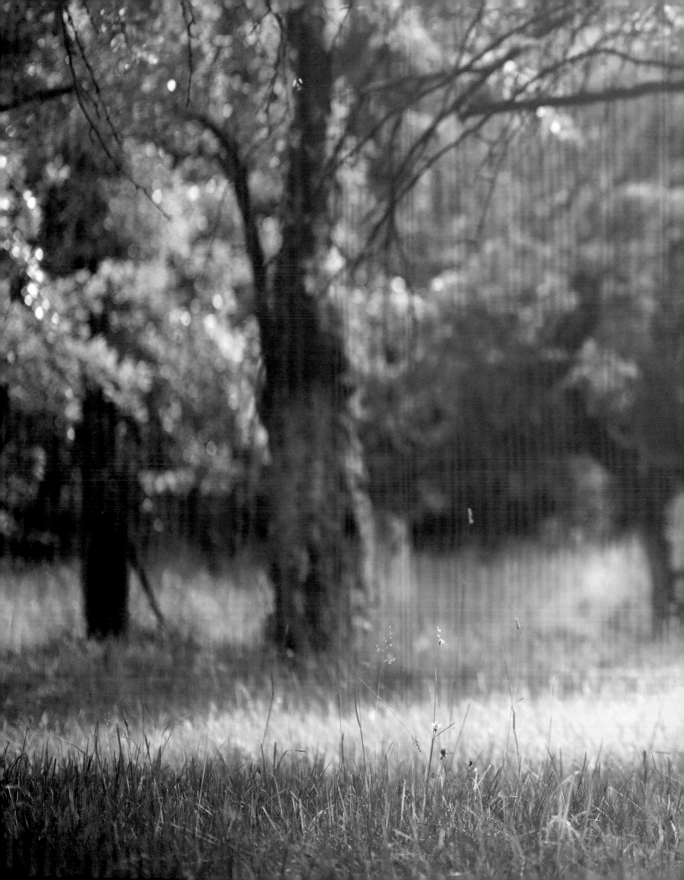

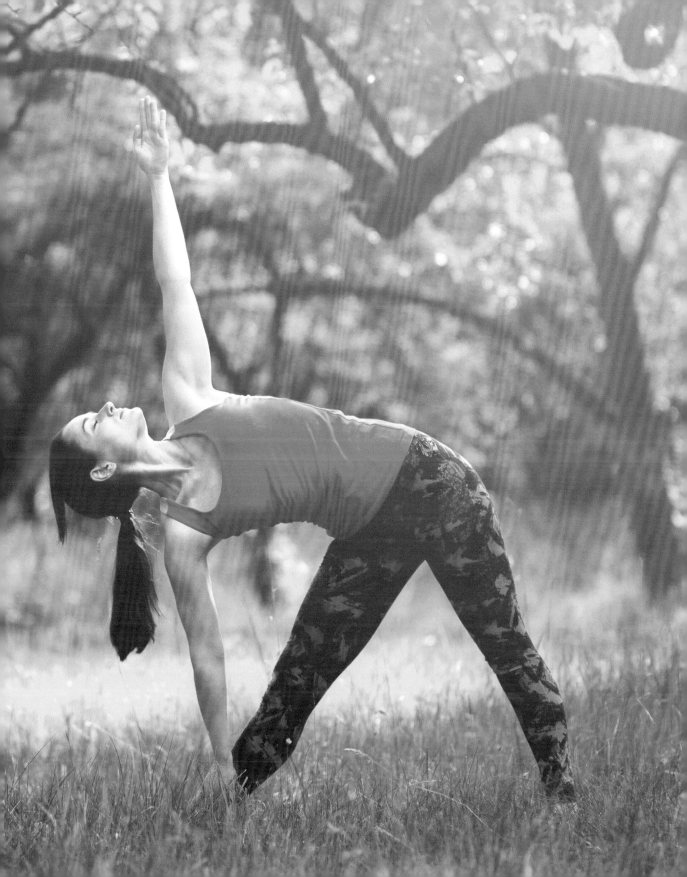

ADHO MUKHA SHVANASANA

Also called the "downward-facing dog", this is a basic inversion pose often practiced as part of the *Surya Namaskar* routine (see pp182–185). It is a great resting pose between two more intense asanas.

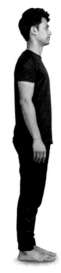

1 Face the shorter edge of the yoga mat. Stand straight with an erect spine. Shoulders and wrists should be aligned so the arm forms a vertical line.

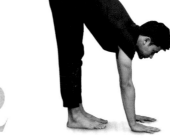

2 Bend at the hips and plant hands on the mat, just beneath the shoulders. On a deep exhalation, slightly bend the knees.

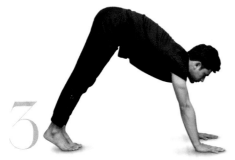

3 Move both legs back one after the other while keeping the weight on the arms. Lift the heels off the ground, keeping the inner arms near the ears. Straighten elbows and knees. Feel the back leg muscles stretch.

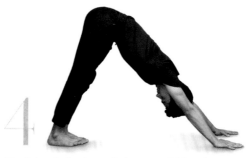

4 Slowly let the heels touch the ground. Fix palms on the mat and push the chest downwards. Look at the feet and inhale deeply.

YOGA ALONE PAVES THE WAY FOR COMPLETE ULTIMATE KNOWLEDGE OF EVERYTHING.

T. KRISHNAMACHARYA, THE "FATHER OF MODERN YOGA"

BAKASANA

This dynamic asana is also known as the "crow pose" as the final posture bears resemblance to the bird. *Bakasana* is essentially an arm balancing pose and challenges the practitioner's core strength. It engages the abdominal muscles and the wrists while fostering deep focus and sense of stability.

BENEFITS & CARE

Bakasana aids concentration and focus, and reduces stress. Do not practise if pregnant, recovering from surgery, or in case of high blood pressure, migraine, or arthritis.

1

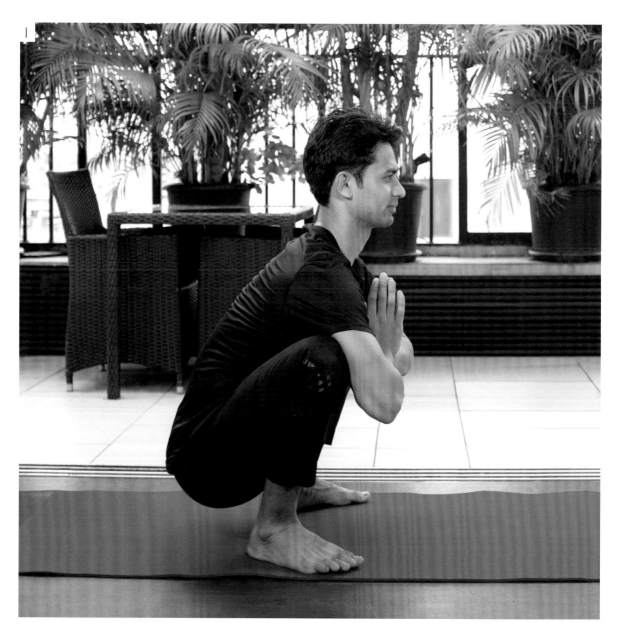

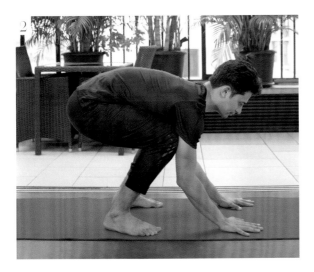

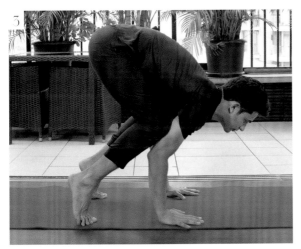

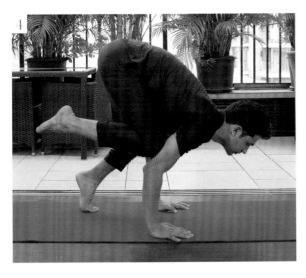

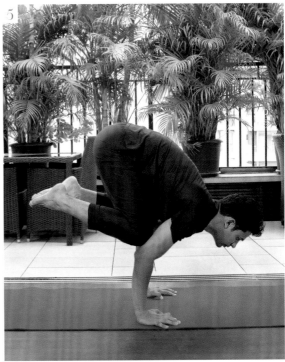

1 Begin in a deep squat or any seated position, facing the shorter edge of the mat. Adjust the hips into a comfortable position before beginning.

2 Place both palms firmly on the mat a little in front of the feet. Spread the fingers and press against the top joints while raising the hips higher.

3 Keep the elbows straight and open the knees so they are parallel to the upper arms. Raise the body up with the weight distributed to the balls of the feet.

4 Stand on the tips of the toes and raise one foot off the ground. Use the inner thighs for support and balance the knees on the upper arms.

5 Slowly lift the other foot off the ground as well so the body is balanced by the arms and knees. Hold for five breaths or more, if comfortable.

SALABHASANA

Salabhasana, also known as the "locust pose", captures the vitality and vigour of a yogi. It involves lifting the legs and chest off the ground in a great stretch. The asana is a good preparatory pose for more rigorous back bends in yoga. Advanced practitioners perform a more complicated version of the pose, but it has been modified here to suit all levels of practitioners.

BENEFITS & CARE

Great for shoulders, hamstrings, back, and glutes. It aids spinal flexibility, improves posture, and reduces stress. Do not attempt if pregnant, or suffering from hernia, high blood pressure, peptic ulcers, arthritis, spinal injury, or heart conditions.

1

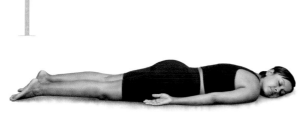

Lie in the prone position with the feet together and arms on either side of the body.

2

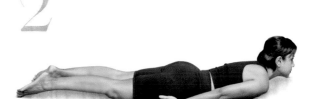

Raise the head upwards by engaging the back, neck, and shoulder muscles. The arms should remain on the ground. Slowly raise the feet off the ground while engaging the thighs and muscles in the lower back.

3

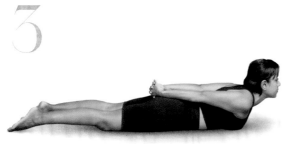

Bring the hands together above the hips and interlock the fingers. Pull the hands backwards and feel the stretch as the arms extend.

4

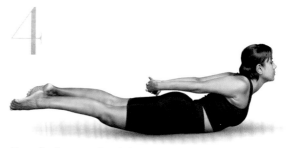

Keep the feet raised and the neck and head lifted and stretch. If interlocking the fingers feels difficult, raise the hands upwards. Hold for five breaths.

USTRASANA

The "camel pose", or *Ustrasana*, resembles the hump of the animal, which gives it its name. This dynamic back-bending asana embodies strength and flexibility as it completely stretches the front of the body, targeting muscles in the chest, abdomen, and hips.

BENEFITS & CARE

Ustrasana tones the body, opens the chest, and improves posture. It also releases emotions and stress. Do not perform if suffering from hernia, knee, shoulder, neck or back injury, or recovering from abdominal surgery.

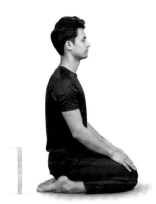

1 Sit on the calves and ankles with the toes pointed backwards and close together. Knees should be slightly separated, but not too much.

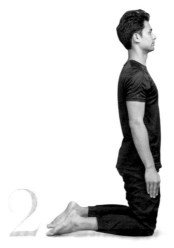

2 Rise up into a kneeling position. Keep the legs parallel to one another and the toes pointed backwards.

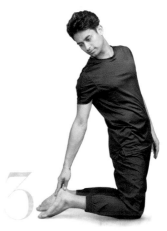

3 Lean back slightly and reach out to hold the left heel with the left hand. Don't exert too much pressure on the knee.

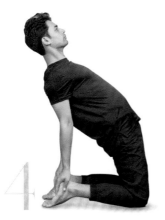

4 Similarly, reach out and hold the right heel with the right hand. Keep thighs vertical and straighten the body. The gaze should be in front.

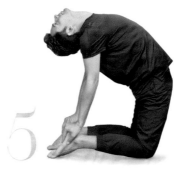

5 Bend back further and curve the spine. Hang the head back and look upwards. There should be no discomfort. Hold the position for five breaths.

SARVANGASANA

The word *Sarvangasana* comprises three Sanskrit words, *sarv* or "all", *anga* or the body's parts, and asana or pose. A foundational posture in yoga, it is also called the "shoulder stand" as the body has to be balanced vertically on the shoulders in the final pose.

BENEFITS & CARE
Targets muscles in the core and upper back, stimulates the thyroid gland, improves posture, enhances mental clarity, and relieves varicose veins. Avoid this pose if suffering from spondylitis, back pain, or spinal injury.

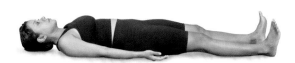

Lie on the back, feet slightly apart and both arms on the ground on either side of the body.

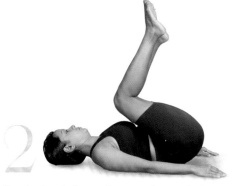

Keeping hands flat on the ground, raise the legs and hips off the ground. Knees can be bent at this stage.

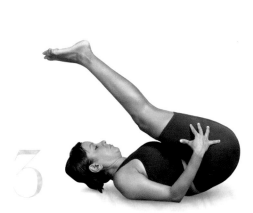

Use the hands to support the hips and extend the legs to the back, straightening the knees.

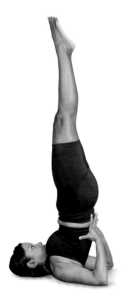

Lift the back and bring both hands to the back for support. Straighten the spine and shift the weight from shoulders to the arms. Hold for 30 seconds or more.

IN FOCUS

Sarvangasana appears like an inverted standing posture resting on the shoulders. As it is an inversion pose, the blood flows towards the practitioner's upper body and head. When one exits the pose, one feels the blood return. This act of inversion brings the practitioner heightened mental clarity and can help focus better, making it a beneficial pose when dealing with mental health issues.

"Yoga allows you to find an inner peace that is not ruffled and riled by the endless stresses and struggles of life."

B.K.S. IYENGAR, FOUNDER OF IYENGAR YOGA

ADHA SIRSASANA

Also known as the "half headstand", the *Adha Sirsasana* is an inversion pose that takes upper body strength to master. It is believed to open up the *sahasrara* chakra, or the crown chakra. This chakra, or energy point, is said to be the centre of higher knowledge, intuition, inspiration, and enlightenment in the body.

BENEFITS & CARE
Adha Sirsasana is great for muscles in the upper body, shoulder, triceps, core, and wrist. It relieves stress, aids balance, and improves concentration. Do not practise this asana if suffering from any injury to the head, neck or spine, high blood pressure, and glaucoma.

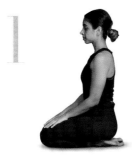

1. Kneel on the ground in *Vajrasana* (see pp122–123). One can place a folded blanket or mat in front.

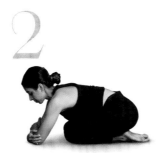

2. Fold the arms and rest them on the ground, or the blanket or mat. Hands should hold the elbows for support.

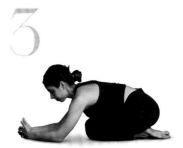

3. Extend the hands in front so that hands are joined and fingers curled in a bowl shape. Continue to kneel.

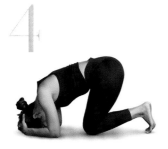

4. Rest the crown of the head in the palms. Raise the hips up from the ground while still touching the ground with the knees.

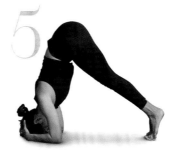

5. Slowly extend the legs and lift the knees as well. Toes should be firmly planted on the ground and the head nestled comfortably in the palms.

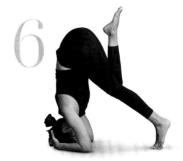

6. Keep the spine parallel to the ground and the right leg straight. Begin to lift the left leg off the ground, while allowing it to bend at the knee.

> "
> It is only when the correct practice is followed for a long time, without interruptions and with a quality of positive attitude and eagerness that it can succeed.
>
> PATANJALI, COMPILER OF *YOGA SUTRAS*, c.401–500 CE
> "

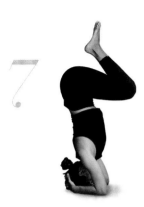

7 Balance the body weight on the arms and try to raise the right leg in the same position as the left. Join both legs together.

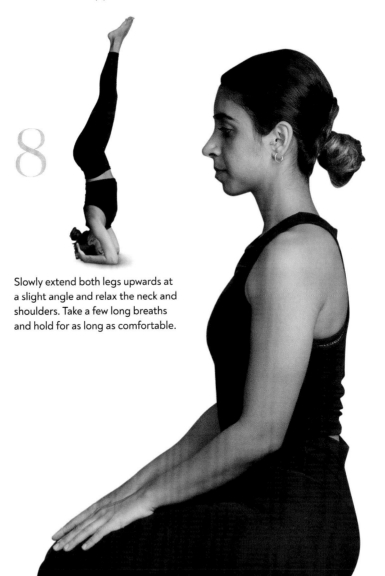

8 Slowly extend both legs upwards at a slight angle and relax the neck and shoulders. Take a few long breaths and hold for as long as comfortable.

9 Take care not to slip or lose balance and slowly return the feet to the ground. To end, sit back in the starting asana, the *Vajrasana* (see pp122–123).

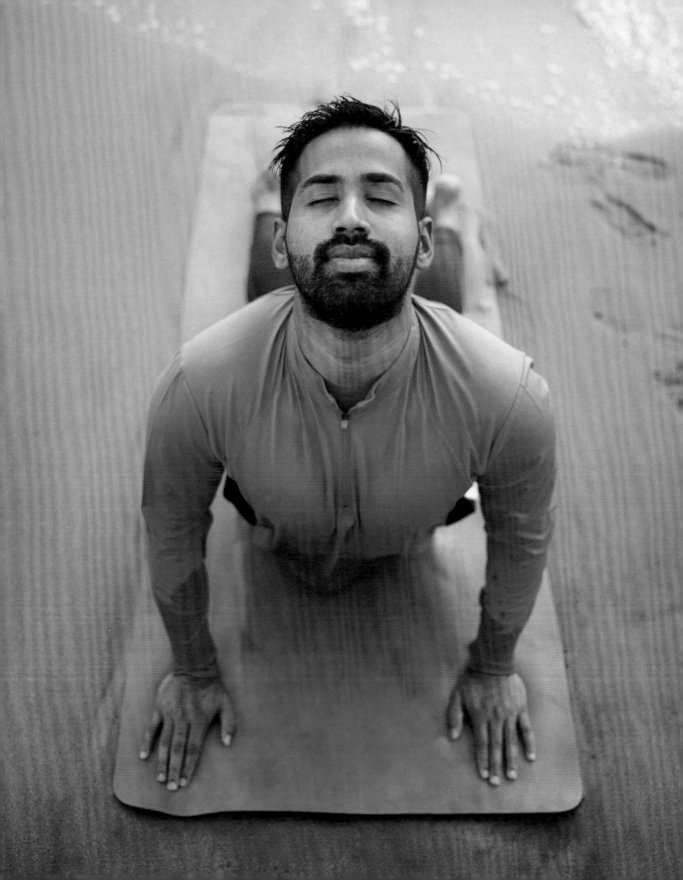

BHUJANGASANA

The "cobra pose", or *Bhujangasana*, is named after the serpent-like position of the body in the final pose. It is a reclining, back-bending asana often performed as part of the *Surya Namaskar* (see pp180–185). It encourages deep breathing and opening of the heart muscles, and fosters a sense of vitality and rejuvenation.

BENEFITS & CARE
Bhujangasana is great for strengthening the back, shoulders, and abdomen. It also relieves weakness, headaches, fatigue, and stress. Those suffering from hernia, ulcers, spondylitis, chronic back or spine pain, recovering from surgery, or those who are pregnant should avoid this asana.

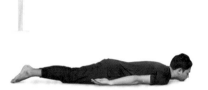

Assume the prone position on the ground. Keep both legs straight and toes together. The arms should be straight on either side of the body.

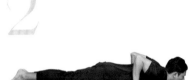

Slide both hands up towards the shoulder with the palms flat on the ground. Doing this will lift and bend the elbows.

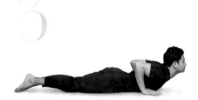

Elevate the upper body by exerting pressure on the palms to lift the torso, neck, and head from the ground.

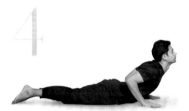

Keep the gaze in front. Put pressure on the hips, thighs, and shoulder blades to achieve a healthy arch of the back and neck.

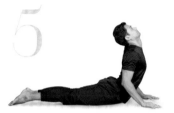

Continue to push upwards and raise the upper body as high as possible without locking the elbows. Hold for five breaths, then release.

IN FOCUS
Through practice of *Bhujangasana*, the adrenal glands and the kidneys are massaged, which aids in functioning. These glands secrete hormones which have vast repercussions on the mind and body. The secretion of adrenaline, for example, regulates the degree of tension and fosters relaxation. This helps bring more stability to the body's mental and physical faculties.

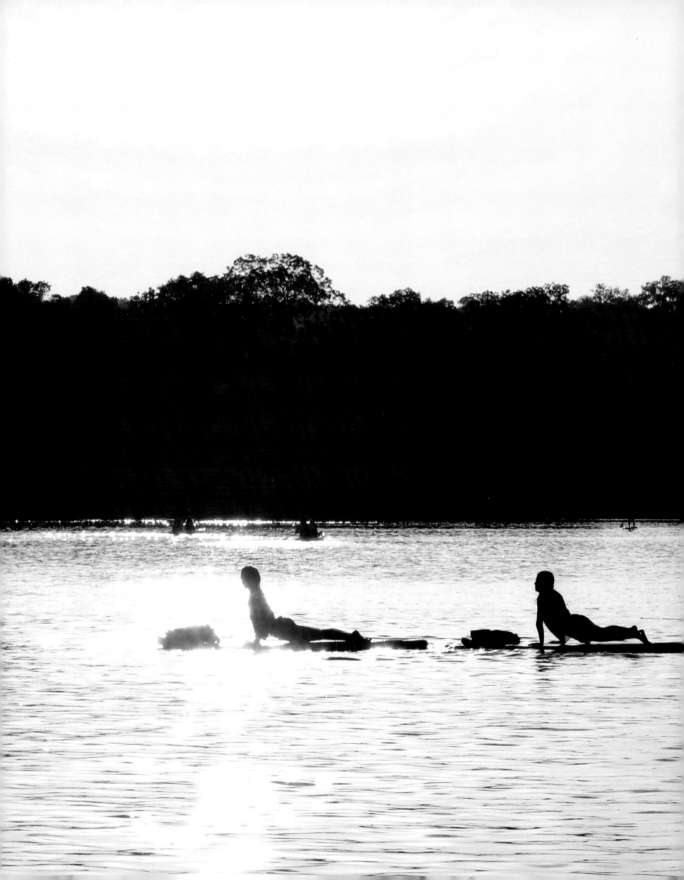

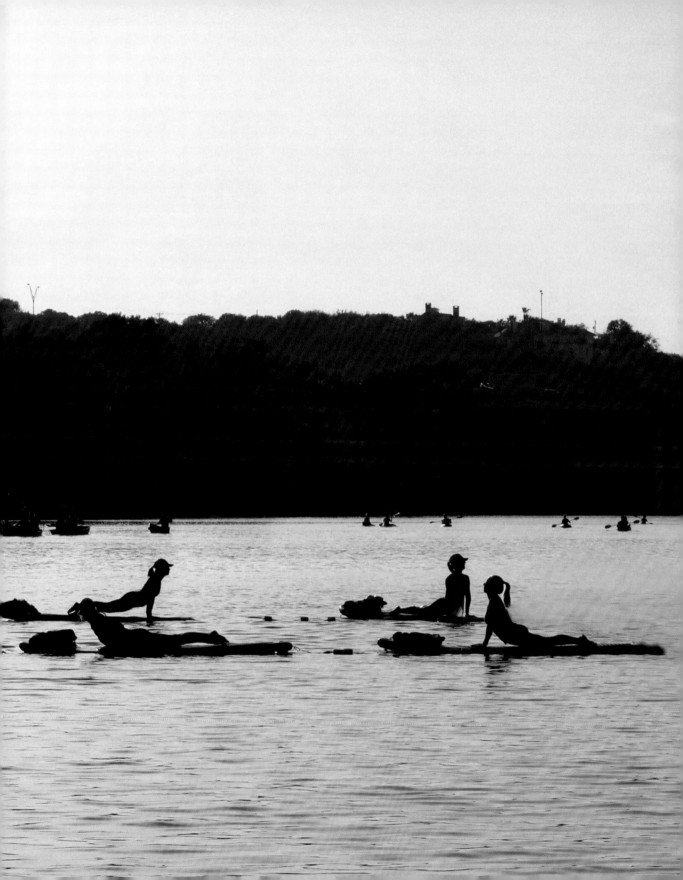

SAVASANA

Often referred to as the "corpse pose" due to the way the body appears in its practice, the *Savasana* is a posture associated with *dhyana*, or meditation. In this resting and restorative position, the practitioner must lie on their back and surrender all thoughts of the past or future. Only then can one achieve the aim of conscious rest.

BENEFITS & CARE

Savasana relieves physical and mental stress from the body by easing fatigue and relaxing the limbs. Regular practice can also ease hypertension and improve sleep. Those who are pregnant, or suffer from chronic back pain or acidity should practise this under supervision, or avoid it.

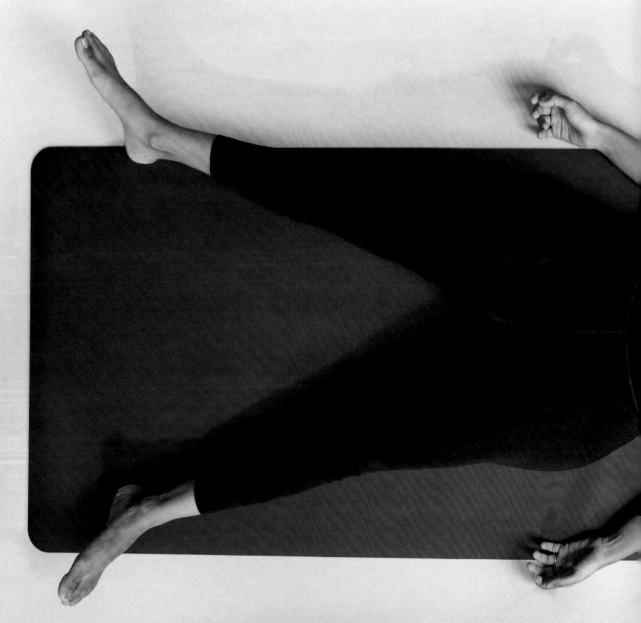

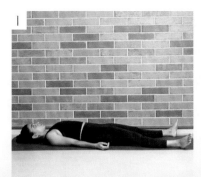

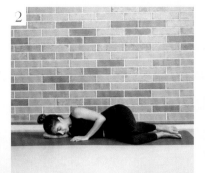

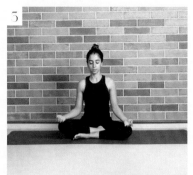

Lie in a supine position with arms at a 15-cm distance from the body and shoulders relaxed. Palms should be turned up and fingertips curled. Close the eyes. Clear the mind, breathe deeply, and remain still. Stay in this position as long as needed.

Become aware of the body slowly, starting from the right foot, the right knee, and continuing to the hip. Repeat with the left leg and continue to think of the body up to the head. Roll to the left and stay in position with the eyes shut. Inhale and exhale slowly.

Gently sit up in a relaxed, cross-legged position, with the help of hands pressing on the ground. Once seated, keep the eyes closed and continue breathing slowly. Rub the palms together and press them to the eye lids, to warm the eyes. Open the eyes slowly.

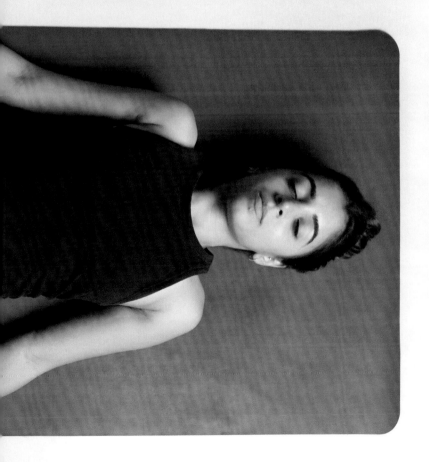

IN FOCUS

Savasana is always performed at the end of a yoga flow or routine. Compared to the other asanas that stimulate the body mentally and physically, the *Savasana* brings quiet and calm to the mind as well as the muscles. Regular practice enables the practitioner to move from an anxious state to one of restoration, where the nervous, immune, and digestive systems are all regulated.

DIRGA PRANAYAMA

Dirga Pranayama, "complete breath", or "three-part breath" is a fundamental pranayama, or breathing technique, that encourages mindful breathing in three distinct parts of the abdomen and lungs. It involves three phases: inhalation, holding the breath, and exhalation. It can be a standalone practice or a foundation for other breathing techniques and meditation.

BENEFITS & CARE

Dirga Pranayama reduces stress, helps in mindfulness, and improves lung capacity and breath control. If pregnant, or having heart, lung, eye, ear problems, or high blood pressure, do not hold the breath in.

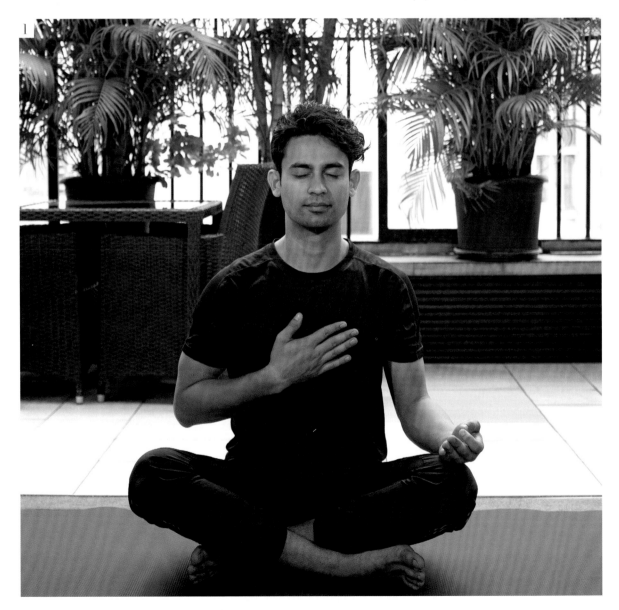

1

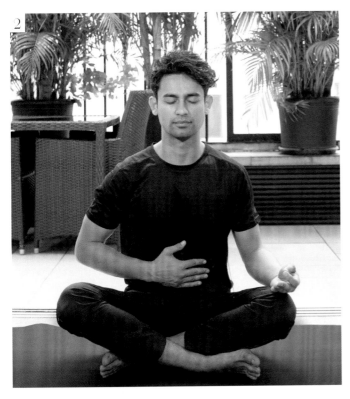

1   Close both eyes and sit comfortably in any cross-legged posture, or in *Sukhasana* (see pp34–35). Start by doing nothing. Only focus on the natural breath of the body while inhaling and exhaling. In case of distractions, bring the focus back to rhythm breathing. Once grounded in the present, start with long and deep breaths. Fill the stomach completely with each inhalation.

2   Place one hand on the belly to feel the inhalation as it expands to fill with air. Perform this deep stomach breathing for five breaths. Then, fill the belly with air again and let it expand into the ribcage. The ribs may feel as though they are spreading. After five breaths, let the air out of the ribcage first, then the stomach and pull the navel back towards the spine.

3   On the next inhalation, fill the gut and ribcage. Place the hand on the heart and feel the area around it rise. Fill it with air up to the collarbone and feel the muscles expand. Hold, and then slowly begin to exhale. Let the breath exit first from the upper chest, letting the heart return to its position, followed by the rib cage as it contracts. Finally, release the air from the stomach and pull the navel back to the spine. Continue breathing in this manner until the transition between the three phases is seamless. Ideally, practise for at least 10 breaths.

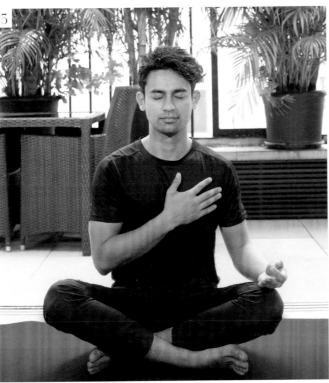

IN FOCUS

Regular practice of this pranayama helps improve one's mental coping ability. It does so by soothing the mind and reducing stress. This helps practitioners improve their quality of sleep. By focusing on the breath for the duration of the asana, the mind is trained to be attentive to the present moment, concentrate on the self, and increase mindfulness.

SINGLE NOSTRIL BREATHING

In yogic practice, the left nostril is associated with cooling energy and the moon, or *chandra*, and the right with heating energy and the sun, or *surya*. The "single nostril breathing" technique involves a deep inhalation using only the left nostril, and exhaling with the right. The practice fosters a sense of calmness and brings down the temperature of the body.

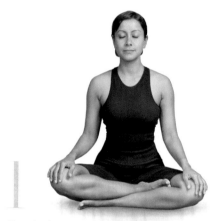

1
Close both eyes and sit in *Sukhasana* (see pp34–35). Keep hands on the knees and relax the body and mind.

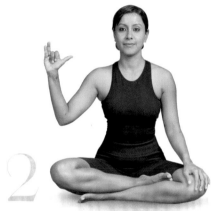

2
Open the eyes and raise one hand. Bring the index and middle fingers together as shown.

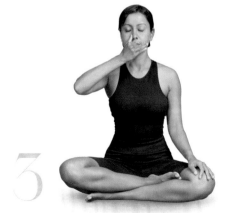

3
Cover the right nostril with the thumb and breathe in through the left. Hold the breath for a few counts.

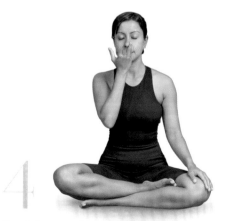

4
To exhale, cover the left nostril with the ring finger and let the breath out using the right nostril. Repeat for as long as comfortable.

TRATAKA

Trataka or "candle gazing" aids in concentration and instilling a sense of stillness. Through this, the disturbances of the mind are dispelled and cognitive functions are improved. Over time, the practice enhances one's ability to manage distractions and cultivates clarity.

BENEFITS & CARE
Trataka strengthens the eye muscles, heightens concentration, and alleviates headaches and fatigue. Do not practise if suffering from glaucoma, high myopia, migraines, or psychological disorders.

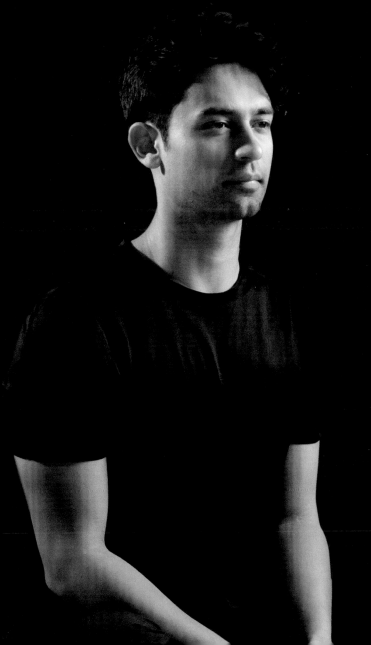

1 Close both eyes and sit in *Sukhasana* (see pp34–35). Keep hands on the knees and relax the body and mind.

2 With the eyes closed, take long, deep breaths through the nose. Aim to exhale for longer than the inhalation.

3 Open the eyes and look directly at the candle's flame. Centre attention to the top of the wick. Don't blink.

4 Let the eyes close naturally when no longer possible to keep open. Keep the candle flame in the mind's eye; it should appear projected in between the eyebrows. When the picture fades, the first round is complete.

DHYANA

Most people are familiar with *dhyana*, or meditation, in at least one of its many forms. Whether through prayer, the act of listening to music, or even careful focus on any task, meditation is all around us. Contrary to popular belief, practising *dhyana* is not about shutting one's thoughts off. It is about focusing on the self and being one with the thoughts, almost as though the self is an observer to them.

BENEFITS & CARE

Dhyana can help decrease fatigue. It increases focus, memory, confidence, and clarity of thoughts. There are no contraindications of meditation, but take care to not strain the body by assuming the posture for too long in the beginning.

1

Prepare the mind to sit motionless for a few minutes. Be comfortable with the body and sit in *Sukhasana* (see pp34–35).

2

Begin by concentrating on the natural breathing motion. Focus on the inhalation and exhalation of the lungs.

3

Feel the breath as it moves through the body – whether it is passing through the nostrils or filling up the stomach.

4

Continue for two minutes. Take a deep breath in and let the stomach expand. Gently exhale, allowing the stomach to compress as the deep breath escapes the body.

5

The goal of meditation is to be thoughtful. Observe the thoughts that come into the mind and gently move them aside, as one would shift a falling leaf from the path.

6

Hold the meditative position for as long as comfortable and possible without distraction. Gradual practice will help increase the duration.

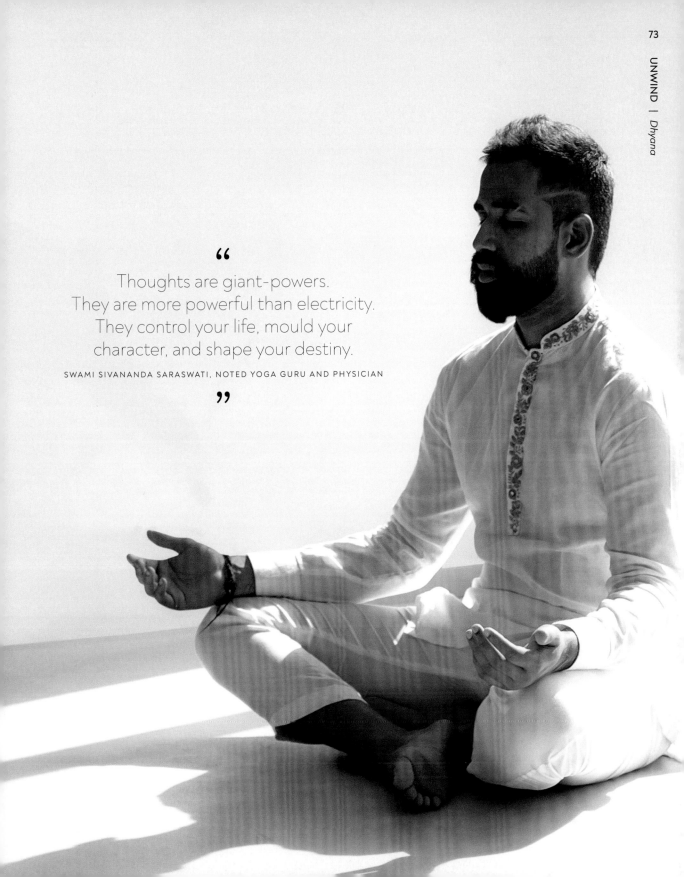

"

Thoughts are giant-powers.
They are more powerful than electricity.
They control your life, mould your
character, and shape your destiny.

SWAMI SIVANANDA SARASWATI, NOTED YOGA GURU AND PHYSICIAN

"

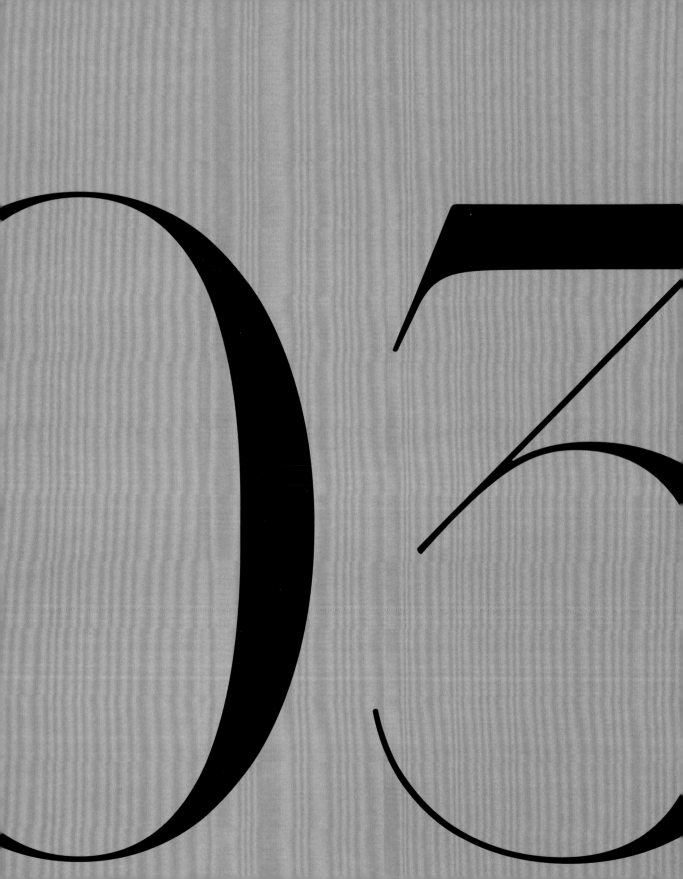

> "
> Yoga allows you to rediscover a sense of wholeness in your life, where you do not feel like you are constantly trying to fit broken pieces together.
>
> B.K.S. IYENGAR, FOUNDER OF IYENGAR YOGA
> "

CALORIE **CRUSHER**

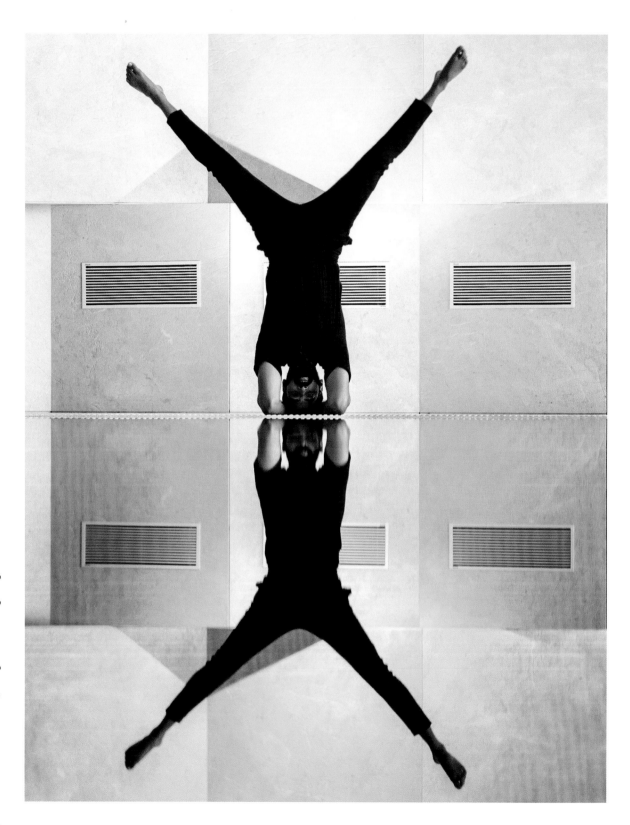

WEIGHT LOSS THROUGH YOGA

Yoga is not just about shedding pounds; it is about finding balance, inner peace, and self-love. The journey to a healthier state begins with embracing the self and appreciating the amazing things our bodies can achieve. Yoga is all about celebrating the body in its current states. It is the support system one needs when embarking on the path to better health.

Dedicated practice helps one build the tools that have an impact on overall wellness. It promotes mindful eating by increasing one's awareness of the food that is consumed and how often. It helps improve sleep patterns, ensuring one wakes up refreshed and energized, which is essential in the weight loss journey.

There are many myths associated with yoga when it comes to losing weight. One I hear often is that yoga can't possibly be intense enough to burn calories. However, if one dives deeper into the practice, one arrives at the realization that yoga is vast and encompasses so much more than the popular perception. Yoga flows increase flexibility, which makes it possible for a person of any body type to engage in. Then there are the yoga holds, or postures where the practitioner utilizes their core to hold for three, five, or more breaths. When one holds, the muscles in the targeted area are activated and the calorie burn is immense. It's similar to how when one holds a plank for a long time one can burn more calories than during a jog. Beyond this, determined and disciplined yogic practice increases metabolism and stamina, enabling for trickier, more intense flows, or other exercises to be incorporated into routines.

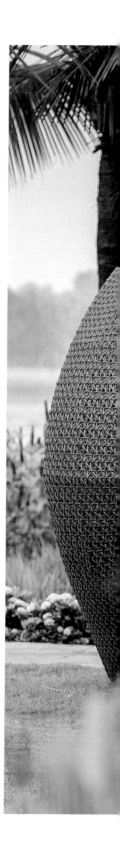

The simplest way to get into regular practice for weight loss is to do the *Surya Namaskar* (see pp180-185) every morning. It is an all-encompassing flow with varied health benefits. Another great asana is the *Adho Mukha Shvanasana* (see pp52-53). It can be coupled with the *Urdhva Mukha Shvanasana* too. Both these postures target muscles in the back, thighs, core, arms, and hamstrings. More experienced practitioners could tailor their routines to include asanas that target the core and the back, such as the *Pawanmuktasana* (see p131) on alternate days for a wholesome sequence

I always urge people to incorporate yoga into their routines even if the primary method of weight management is different. Through yoga, one can lower cortisol levels, improve digestion, and so much more. I've seen it transform my mother's life over the last few years, when medical concerns left her in pain and knee problems led to a life without much exercise. I helped her adjust her diet and worked on a simple yogic flow for her that didn't put much pressure on her knees. In four months, she lost 22kg (48.5lbs).

It is a matter of being consistent with the practice and the movement. It doesn't need to be intense exercise from the beginning. Start with 10 minutes a day, which is enough time for six sets of *Surya Namaskars* every morning. An important step in order to gain most out of yoga is to eat an early and light dinner. This will help with the yoga flow the next day. The goal is simple, really: to take time out for one's self every day, without fail, no matter how busy life gets.

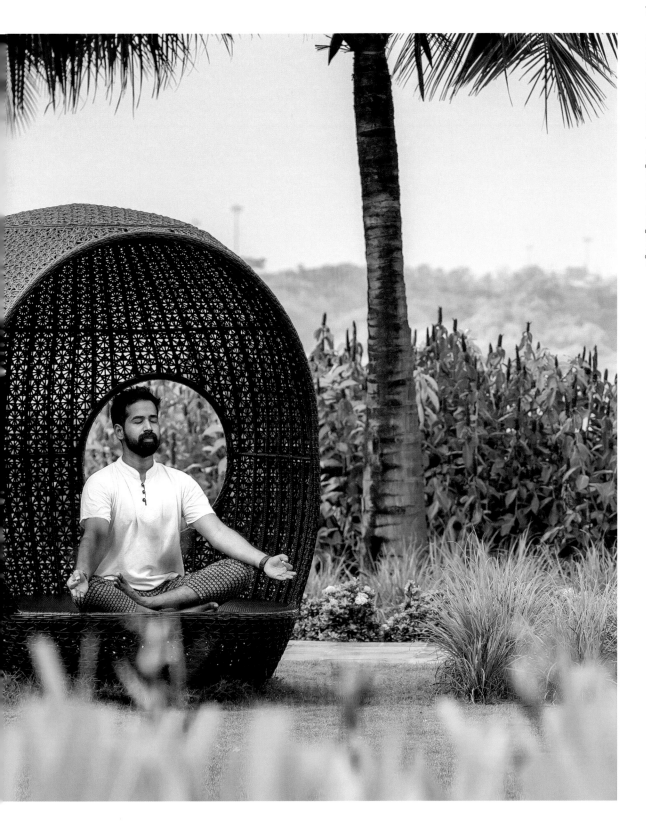

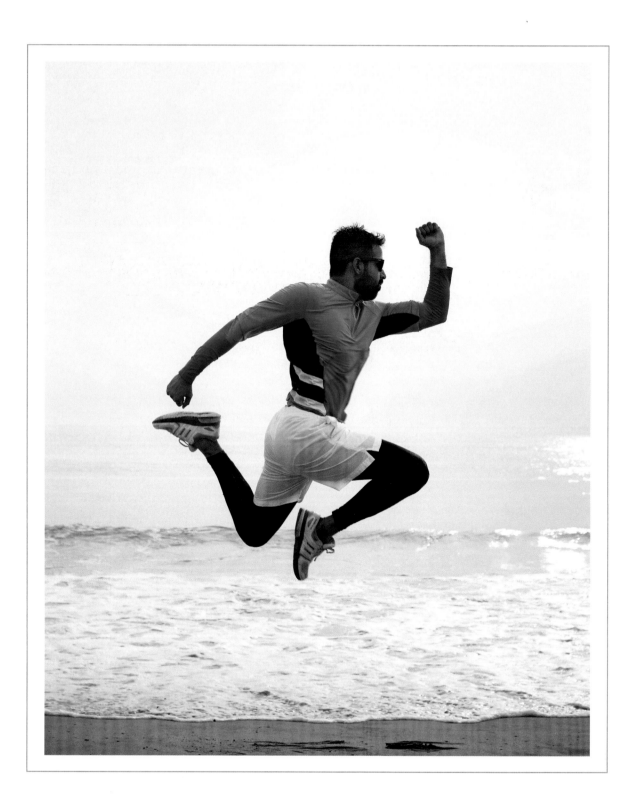

MOVE for five minutes every day. The best way to do that in yoga is by performing the *Surya Namaskar*, or "sun salutation". This daily movement activates your muscles and brings balance to the body and peace to the mind. Treat each asana within the entire flow as an intentional union of the body's limits and capabilities. Moving can also include walking, jogging, or running, if you so wish, but whatever you do, you must be disciplined and deliberate in your approach. Move regularly for a week and you will see the difference.

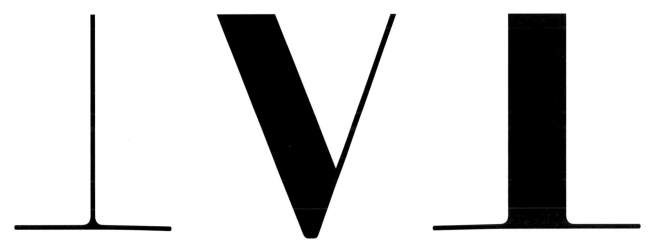

CALORIE CRUSHER FLOW

Research on yoga shows that it can help with weight management through dedicated routines that target the right areas of the body as well as stimulate the mind. From *Sukhasana* (see p84) to *Anulom Vilom* (see p109) and *Dhyana* (see pp72–73), the asanas in this sequence will help manage stress, regulate emotions, burn calories, and even tone muscles. Regular practice can reduce joint and muscle pains which will enable more rigorous exercise.

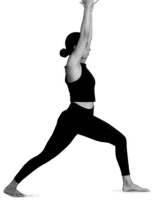

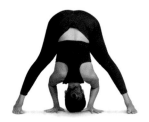

5 **Parsarita Padottanasana**
Page 90

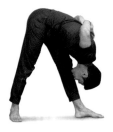

6 **Parsvottanasana**
Page 91

7 **Virabhadrasana I**
Pages 92–93

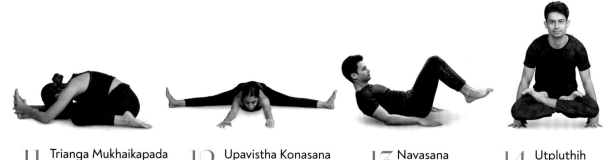

11 **Trianga Mukhaikapada Paschimottanasana**
Pages 100–101

12 **Upavistha Konasana**
Pages 102–103

13 **Navasana**
Pages 104–105

14 **Utpluthih**
Page 106

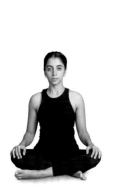

1 Sukhasana
Page 84

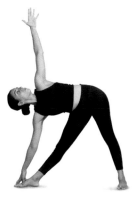

2 Trikonasana
Page 85

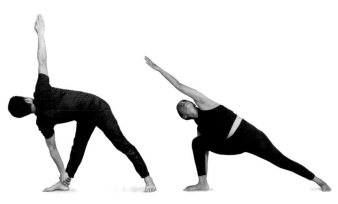

3 Parivrtta Trikonasana
Page 86

4 Utthita Parsvakonasana
Page 87

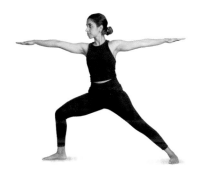

8 Virabhadrasana II
Pages 94–95

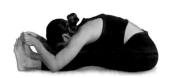

9 Paschimottanasana
Pages 96–97

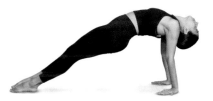

10 Purvottanasana
Page 98–99

It is impactful to end every yoga flow or routine with a few moments of meditation. This is beneficial in bringing the mind and body back to a regulated sense of calm. Dedicated practice brings about a good understanding of the self, including fostering a better relationship with food, the body, and exercise.

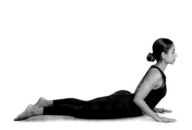

15 Bhujangasana
Page 107

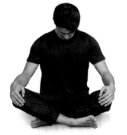

16 Jalandhar Bandha
Page 108

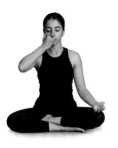

17 Anulom Vilom
Page 109

18 Dhyana
Pages 72–73

SUKHASANA

As its name indicates, the "easy sitting" pose, or *Sukhasana*, is a foundational seated pose in any meditative practice. The final posture of the asana should be maintained as long as comfortable to help strengthen the hip and back.

BENEFITS & CARE

Sukhasana promotes relaxation and helps in meditation and breathing. It eases lower back and knee pain. Avoid it in case of previous knee or hip injuries, or any chronic knee or back pain.

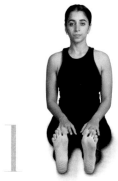

Sit with both legs stretched out in front. The neck and back should remain straight at all times.

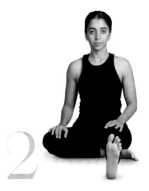

Keep the spine straight, fold the right leg at the knee, and bring the sole of the foot to rest under the other thigh.

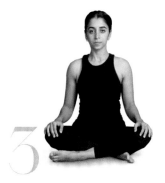

Repeat the same movement with the left leg and adjust the seating position so as to feel minimal pressure on both ankles.

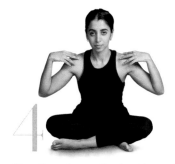

Place the palms on the shoulders and gently move the shoulder back to its original resting position. Keep the head raised and the crown facing up.

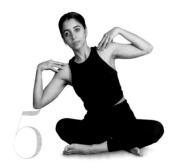

Maintaining the position of the head, move side to side. Breathe normally. Repeat as many times as needed to feel "loose" enough to begin other asanas.

IN FOCUS

In this flow, the folded-leg posture and straight back enables blood flow towards the centre of the body. Yogic wisdom emphasizes sitting in this asana when eating meals as well. The posture improves the digestive functioning of the body, which can reduce bloating and water retention, thus supporting weight loss.

TRIKONASANA

The "three-angles", or "triangle pose", also called the *Trikonasana*, embodies balance and expansion. It is a great stretching posture that strengthens the legs and improves flexibility, making it a good foundation for more rigorous yoga routines.

BENEFITS & CARE

This strengthens muscles in the legs, hips, back, shoulders, and chest. Those with previous neck and back injuries, chronic migraine, or blood pressure issues should take care when performing the asana or avoid it.

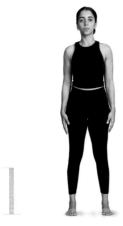

1 Stand with feet three-feet apart and hands straight next to the hips. The space between the feet may be adapted to what is comfortable, as per one's height.

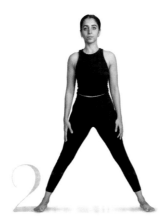

2 Slowly turn the right foot outwards at a 90-degree angle to the left foot. Maintain the gaze at an object at eye level, and stay balanced.

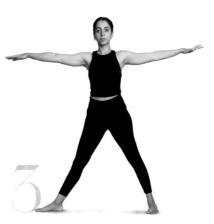

3 Raise arms until parallel to the floor and in line with each other. Bend to the side and reach for the right ankle with the right hand.

4 In the final pose, the right hand is on the right ankle, the left hand is raised to the sky, and the gaze is upwards, set upon the left palm.

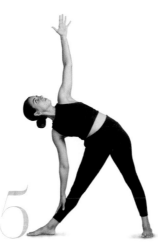

5 The body must not droop forwards and arms must be taut for an intense stretch on the side. If needed, place hand on the shin. Repeat the same on the other side.

IN FOCUS

Within the weight loss flow, the *Trikonasana* is one of the easiest asanas to master. As a side-bending pose, it fosters a deep stretch on both the sides, essentially massaging the tissues and muscles in the waist. This posture helps with toning the sides, which aids in overall weight loss.

PARIVRTTA TRIKONASANA

BENEFITS & CARE

The asana enhances flexibility and balance, and strengthens legs and spine. Those who are pregnant, or have neck or spine injuries, back pain, migraines, low blood pressure, or diarrhoea should avoid *Parivrtta Trikonasana*.

Also called the "revolved triangle pose", this variation of the *Trikonasana* involves spinal rotation. In this pose, the practitioner twists their torso, reaching down to touch the feet. This asana also has many benefits for spinal flexibility and strength.

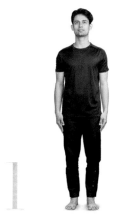

1 Stand straight and place both hands alongside the hips, with the arms straight. Find a position that is comfortable and relax the body.

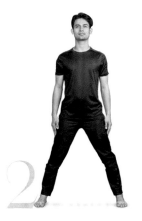

2 Spread feet three-feet apart or to what is comfortable. Hands should remain at the sides. Try to square the hips and feel the weight collect at the feet.

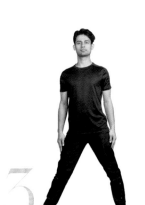

3 Angle the right foot outwards at a 90-degree angle to earlier. Shift the body weight to the left foot for balance.

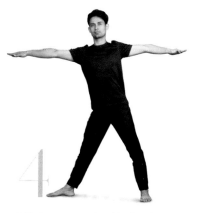

4 Lift the arms to shoulder height and extend, keeping them parallel to the ground. Keep the body balanced and look to the front.

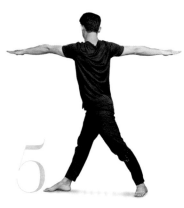

5 Rotate the torso such that the left hand is parallel to the right foot and vice versa. Hold this position for five breaths.

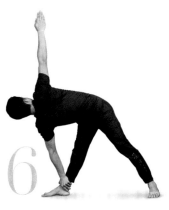

6 Bend down to reach for the right ankle, or shin, with the left hand. This is the final pose. Hold for five breaths and repeat on the other side.

UTTHITA PARSVAKONASANA

Utthita Parsvakonasana, or the "extended side angle pose", is named after the extended angle formed as the practitioner performs it. This empowering asana intensifies the stretch of the more simple *Parsvakonasana* while promoting a sense of stability and openness.

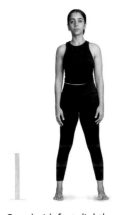

Stand with feet slightly apart and place both hands alongside the hips. Relax the body to prepare for the asana.

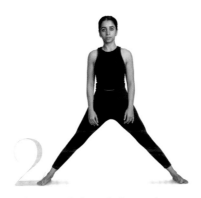

Side step with the right foot and spread the legs as much as possible. Hands should be relaxed but can be placed on the hips for balance.

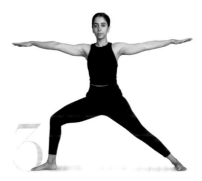

Turn the right foot outwards at a 90-degree angle. Raise both hands and extend them parallel to the ground. Bend the right knee slightly.

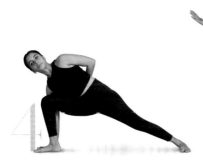

Exhale and bend the body over the right leg. Touch the ground with the right hand, placing it on the inside or outside of the foot. Move left hand to the back.

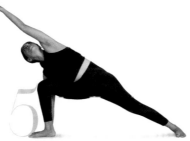

Extend the left hand over the head, parallel to the ear, palm facing down. Turn gaze to the hand. Hold this position for five breaths.

BENEFITS & CARE

Utthita Parsvakonasana tones ankles and thighs. Regular practice improves digestion and reduces waist and hip fat. Those with irregular blood pressure, or neck, knee, or shoulder injury should avoid.

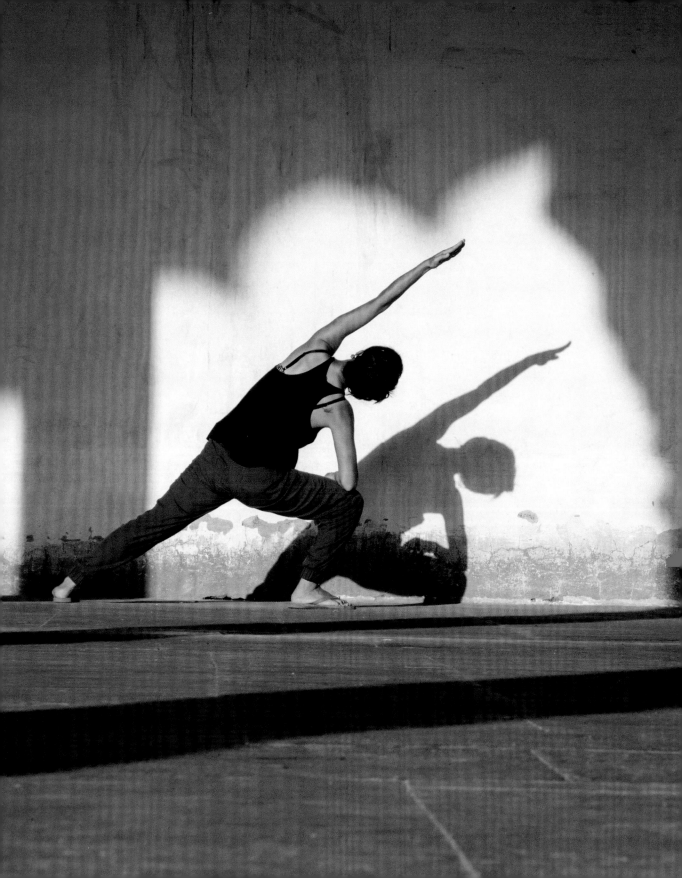

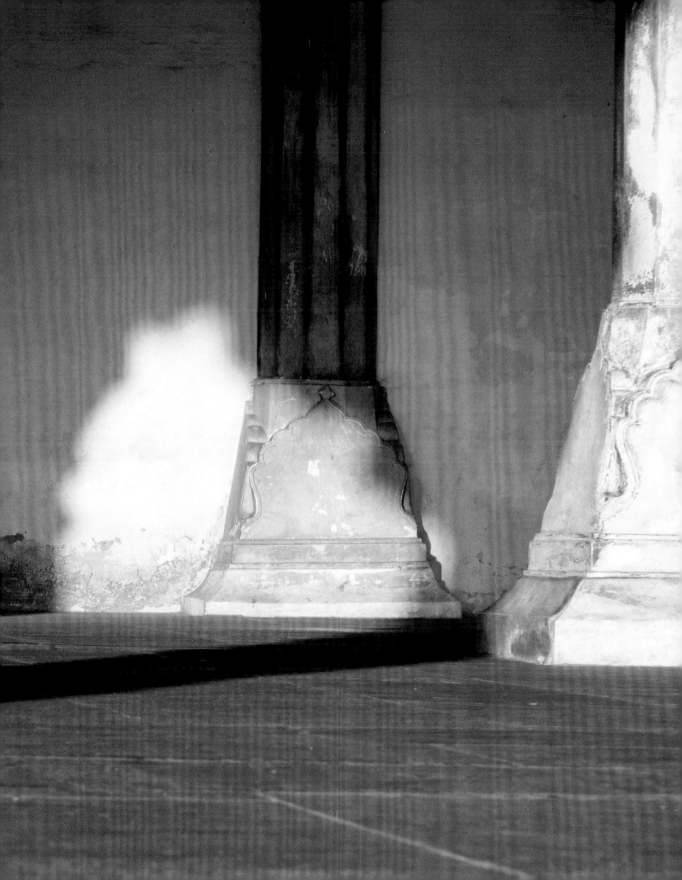

PARSARITA PADOTTANASANA

This asana, also called the "wide-legged forward bend", is, as the name suggests, a deep forward fold of the body. In this pose, the legs are wide apart, the torso is completely lowered, hinging at the hips. It is a great grounding asana for achieving flexibility.

BENEFITS & CARE

This is a good asana for concentration, and for toning muscles in the legs, chest, and arms. Those with neck, spine, or shoulder injuries, or vertigo, glaucoma, or heart conditions should avoid this.

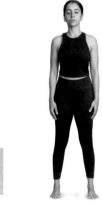

1 Stand with the arms resting straight on either side, against the hips and the legs slightly apart. Relax the body.

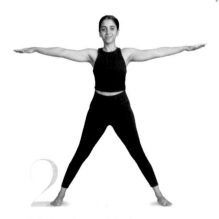

2 Exhale and spread the legs, but not too wide. Raise both arms and extend parallel to the ground.

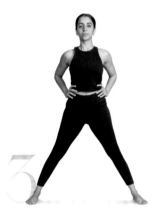

3 Bring the hands down with palms resting on the hips. The posture should be erect and spine extended.

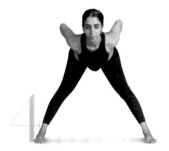

4 Bend forwards at the hips so that the upper body is parallel to the ground. Ensure that the gaze is straight ahead.

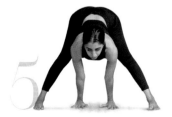

5 Lower both hands and touch the ground with the fingers, then palms. Let the elbows fold back as the body is lowered further.

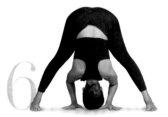

6 Try to bring the head down so that the crown touches the ground, or as close as possible. Stay in this position for five breaths, then gently release and rise up.

PARSVOTTANASANA

The "pyramid pose", as this is also known, highlights the practitioner's strength and balance. In the final pose, the body resembles a pyramid, with the torso folding to the side completely, hinged at the hips. *Parsvottanasana* symbolizes the alignment of the body and encourages physical and mental poise.

BENEFITS & CARE

Parsvottanasana stretches the hamstrings and calves, fosters stability in the back and legs, and improves digestion. Avoid it in case of chronic pain or injury to the hips, back, or shoulders.

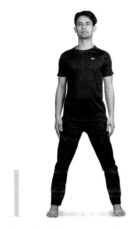

1 Stand with the arms resting straight on either side, against the hips and the legs shoulder-width apart. Relax the body.

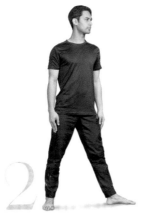

2 Turn the left foot outwards at a 90-degree angle. Simultaneously turn the upper body towards the left leg.

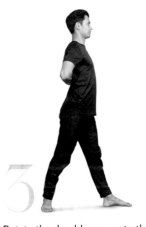

3 Rotate the shoulders more to the left. Fold the arms at the back and join hands in a reverse prayer position. The chest should feel open, and the spine straight.

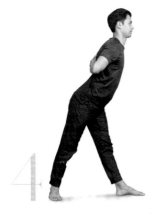

4 On an exhalation, begin to push the chest downward and bend forwards at the hips. The head should be straight and gaze in front.

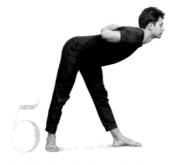

5 Push the hips back to maintain a squared pelvis. Try to bring the stomach in and continue to bend forwards with the spine straight.

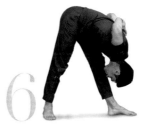

6 Bend the head and continue. Touch the stomach to the thighs and chest to legs. If needed, raise the hands up instead of the prayer position.

MASTER YOUR BREATH AND LET THE SELF BE IN BLISS. CONTEMPLATE ON THE SUBLIME WITHIN YOU.

T. KRISHNAMACHARYA, THE "FATHER OF MODERN YOGA"

VIRABHADRASANA I

Also called "Warrior I", this foundational asana embodies the strength, determination, and readiness of a warrior, giving it its name. In this asana, one foot is extended in front while the other remains straight at the back. The arms reach up to the sky in a great stretch of the torso.

BENEFITS & CARE

Virabhadrasana I fosters mental strength, improves air circulation, activates abdominal muscles, and regulates digestion. Those who are pregnant, or have hip, knee, shoulder or back injuries should avoid Warrior I.

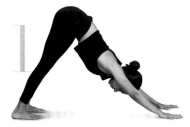

Start in *Adho Mukha Shvanasana* (see p52) with the hips raised and the body forming a triangle.

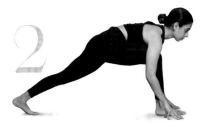

Bring the left foot forwards so that the toes are in line with the fingers. Shift the foot slightly to the left. Hips should be lowered and the head straightened.

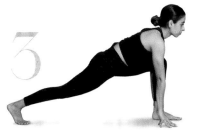

Bend the left knee and stretch the right leg back till it rests on the toes. The knee should be in line with the ankle and the left outer hip should be pinned back.

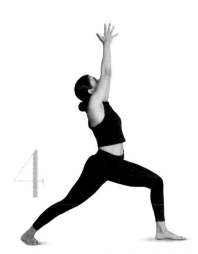

Lift the torso up until upright, raise both arms, palms facing each other. Inhale and let the shoulder blades expand up and outwards, away from the spine.

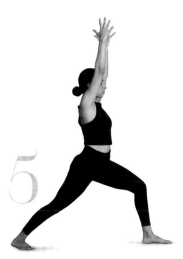

Gaze should be set at the thumbs but can be straight ahead. Hold the pose for five breaths. Return to the starting position and repeat on the other side.

IN FOCUS

In this particular flow, this asana, *Virabhadrasana I*, is effective in burning calories, losing abdominal fat and toning muscles. It is why this is a staple of any weight loss flow. The deep stretch strengthens muscles in the thigh, lower back, and pelvis. Regular practice can help to improve metabolism by targeting the core and practitioners may see inch loss around the hips.

VIRABHADRASANA II

The "Warrior II" is a dynamic asana characterized by a wide-legged stance that embodies the strength and grace of a warrior. It is a foundational yoga pose that targets several muscle groups and provides a deep and invigorating stretch. This is a variation on the asana discussed in the previous chapter (see pp46–47).

BENEFITS & CARE

Virabhadrasana II impacts thighs, hips, glutes, quadriceps, and shoulders. It improves balance, posture, flexibility, and reduces stress and relieves stores tension. Those with recent or chronic injury to the hips, knees, or shoulders should avoid the asana.

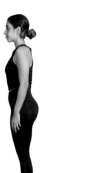

1

Stand facing the shorter side of the mat with both feet parallel to one another.

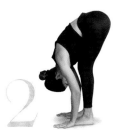

2

Bend forwards and support the body weight by applying equal pressure on the hands where they are placed on the ground.

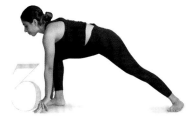

3

Shift the weight on the right leg and take a big step back with the left. Point the left toes outwards, straighten the spine, and keep the gaze fixed in front.

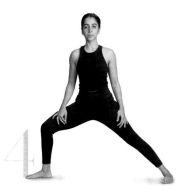

4

Extend the right knee and bring it into a vertical line with the ankle. Straighten the spine, face in front, and equally distribute the weight on both legs.

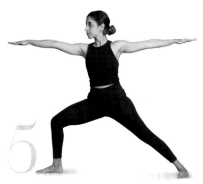

5

Raise both hands parallel to the ground and turn the head towards the right hand. The spine should be straight. Hold the pose for five breaths.

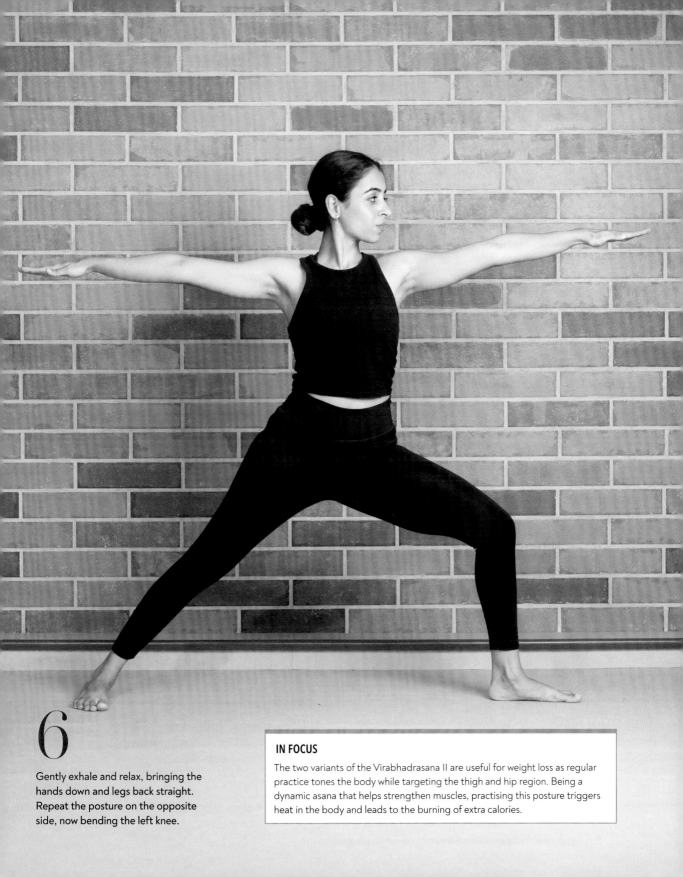

6

Gently exhale and relax, bringing the hands down and legs back straight. Repeat the posture on the opposite side, now bending the left knee.

IN FOCUS

The two variants of the Virabhadrasana II are useful for weight loss as regular practice tones the body while targeting the thigh and hip region. Being a dynamic asana that helps strengthen muscles, practising this posture triggers heat in the body and leads to the burning of extra calories.

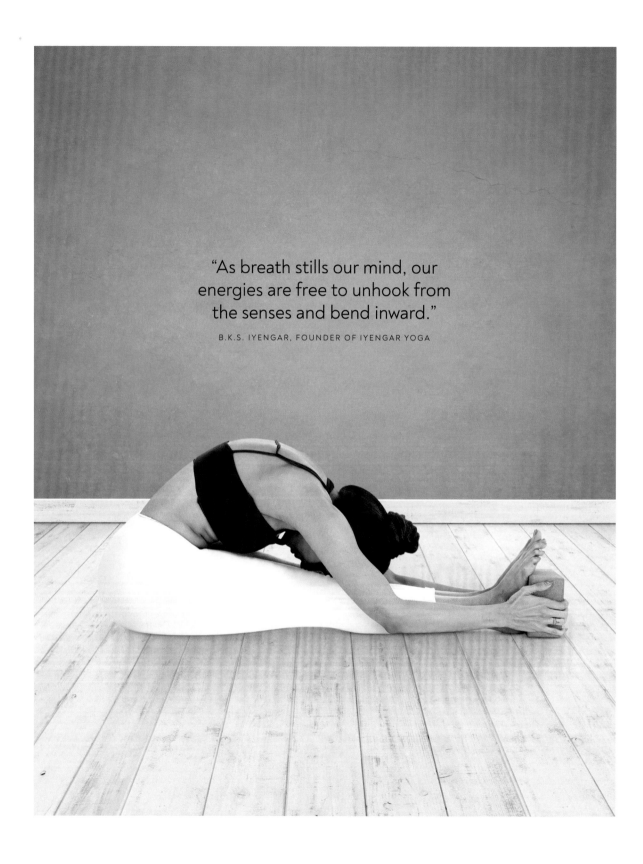

"As breath stills our mind, our energies are free to unhook from the senses and bend inward."

B.K.S. IYENGAR, FOUNDER OF IYENGAR YOGA

PASCHIMOTTANASANA

The "seated forward bend", or *Paschimottanasana*, as the name suggests, is a deep forward fold of the upper body in seated position. In the final pose, the entire torso is folded over the legs, with the hands holding the big toes. In yoga, this symbolizes introspection and surrender, offering a sense of calm and release from stress.

BENEFITS & CARE

Regular practice stimulates the nervous system, tones the shoulder, back, arm and legs, and reduces fat from the abdomen and thighs. Avoid in case of lower back or neck injury, high blood pressure, glaucoma, slip disc, hernia, or pregnancy.

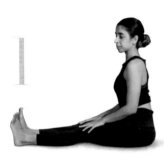

Sit on the ground with the spine upright. Extend the legs in front, but do not let them touch. Inhale deeply and let the chest expand.

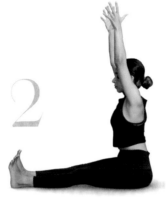

Raise both arms up and continue to breathe deeply. The head should be straight, spine extended, and gaze in front.

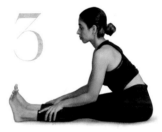

Lean forwards to grip the feet. Try to keep the hips in position and the spine straight.

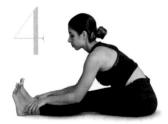

Lean forwards slowly, as the hands inch down the legs and towards the ankles. The back should not be rounded when doing this.

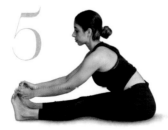

Try and grasp the big toes with the fingers. Keep the back straight. If that is not possible, reach the furthest spot whether it is the calves or the ankles.

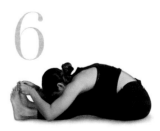

Lower the head to touch the legs with the forehead. If not possible, bring as close to the body as is comfortable. Hold the pose for five breaths.

PURVOTTANASANA

Purvottanasana, the "upward plank" or "reverse plank", is an empowering balancing asana that is all about the expansion of the body and building strength. The name roughly translates to "intense eastern stretch". The asana symbolizes rejuvenation and openness of emotions and is considered an energizing pose.

BENEFITS & CARE

Great for engaging the abdomen, toning stomach, better respiratory function, and stress relief. Avoid it if pregnant, suffering from migraine, high blood pressure, any injuries, or if on an empty stomach.

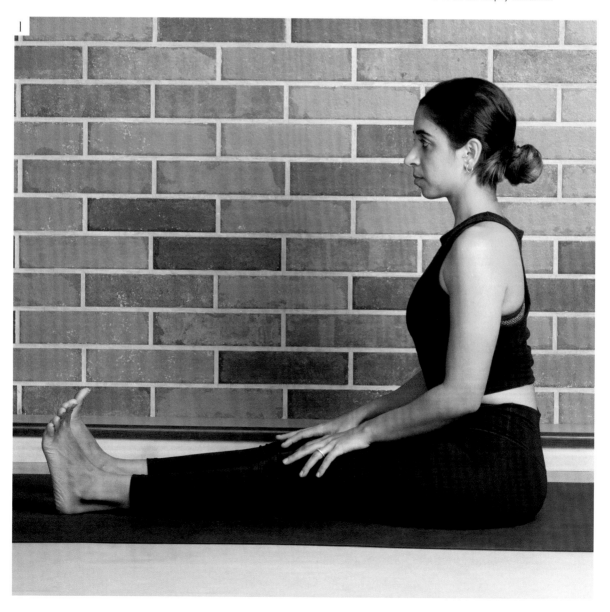

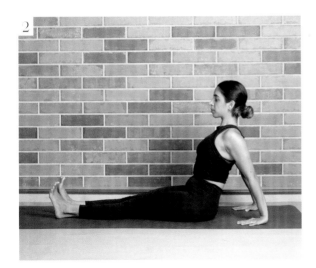

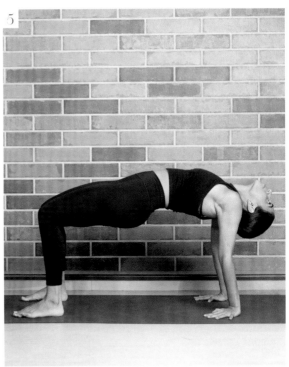

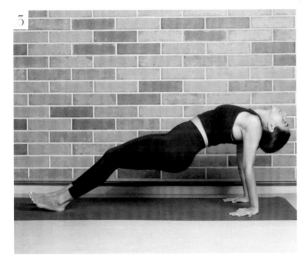

1 Sit with the back straight and legs stretched out in front. Hands should rest on the thighs and the head should also be facing the front.

2 Draw the arms backwards and place the hands on the mat behind the hips. Palms should touch the ground with the fingers pointing towards the hips.

3 Raise the body up, heels touching the ground. Ensure that the weight is distributed upon the hands and feet.

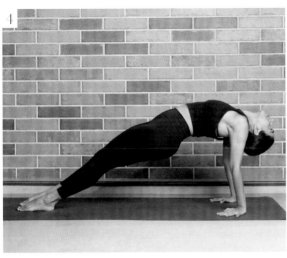

4 Exhale and lift the hips higher, in line with the shoulders, so the body rests in an inverted table-top position. Flatten the toes and plant hand and feet firmly on the ground. Hold for five breaths.

5 If needed, relax the pose to bend the legs at the knees and hold this position as long as possible.

TRIANGA MUKHAIKAPADA PASCHIMOTTANASANA

Also called the "one-legged forward bend in three parts" or the "three-limbed intense west stretch", this challenging yoga posture combines elements of forward folding and leg extension. In the final asana, one leg is stretched straight in front, while the other is bent at the knee, and the body is folded completely over the legs.

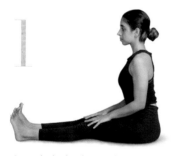

Sit with the back straight and legs stretched out in front. Hands should rest on the thighs and the head should also be facing the front.

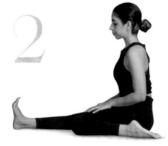

Bending the knee, fold the left leg and place the foot next to the left hip. The inner calf muscles and the outside of the thigh should be touching.

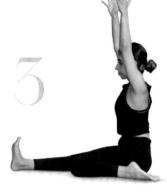

Relax the shoulders and find the balance. On a deep inhalation, slowly raise the arms above the head, but do not join hands.

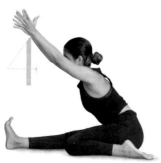

Exhale and slowly bend forwards. The spine should remain erect, and the arms straight as the body moves forwards.

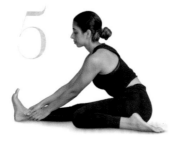

Reach down with the arms and hold the ankle of the right foot in both hands. Keep the back straight.

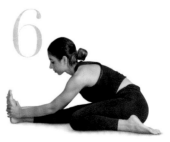

Lower the torso more so that the stomach touches the thighs and the forearm lays flat against the leg.

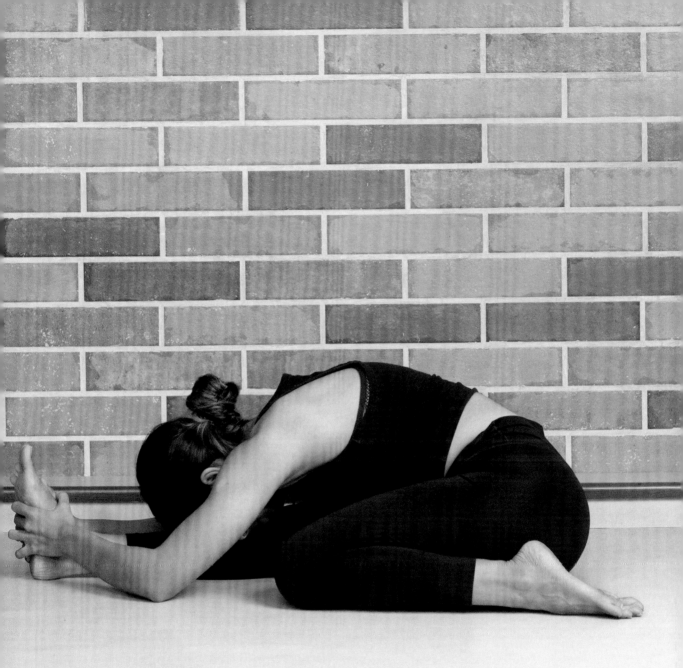

7

Touch the head and the nose to the leg.
Place the chin on the shin and hold the
position for five breaths. Relax the body,
sit upright, and repeat the posture on
the other side, folding the right leg.

BENEFITS & CARE

Trianga Mukhaikapada Paschimottanasana
stimulates the muscles in the abdomen, back,
and pelvis, and regulates stomach, kidney,
and liver functions. It also helps with sciatica,
piriformis syndrome, and plantar fasciitis. Those
who are pregnant or have a weak digestive
system, and those with wrist, knee, hip, and
shoulder injuries should avoid this asana.

UPAVISTHA KONASANA

The *Upavistha Konasana* is a seated forward fold of the torso, practiced with the legs stretched wide in a straight line. This deep stretch targets muscles on the inner thighs, groins, and hamstrings, while enhancing flexibility and calming the mind. Symbolically, it speaks to introspection and openness, and its practice offers release and sense of tranquillity.

BENEFITS & CARE

Upavistha Konasana is great for activating joints and muscles in the groin and abdomen. It also enhances spinal flexibility and relieves sciatica and arthritis pain, fatigue, and anxiety. Don't practise this if pregnant, suffering from hip, back, or wrist injury, or slipped disc.

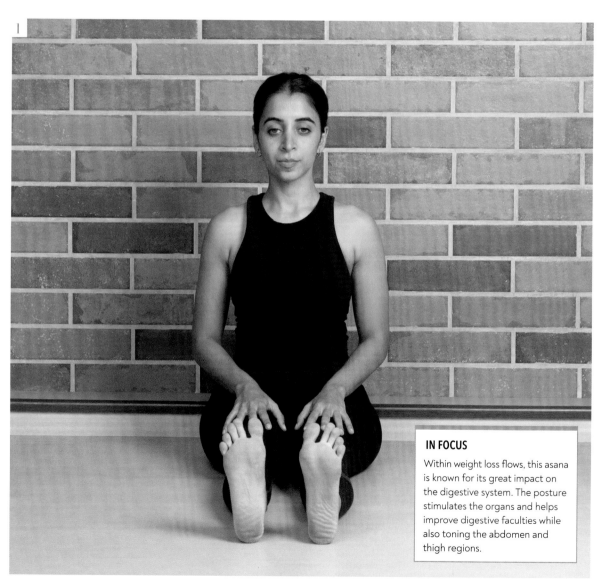

IN FOCUS

Within weight loss flows, this asana is known for its great impact on the digestive system. The posture stimulates the organs and helps improve digestive faculties while also toning the abdomen and thigh regions.

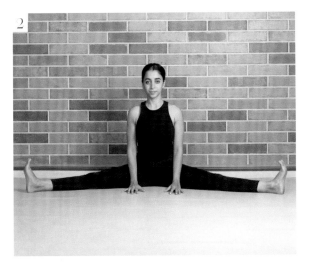

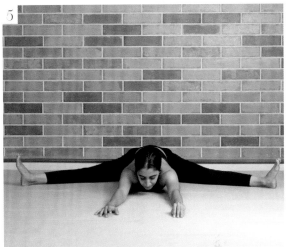

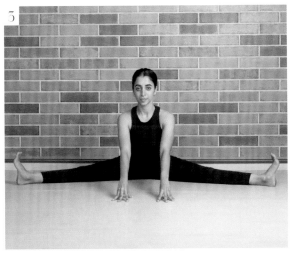

1 Sit with the back straight and legs stretched out in front. Toes should point up, hands should rest on the thighs, and the head should face the front.

2 Spread the legs as wide as possible. Ideally, the legs should be positioned at a 90-degree angle to the pelvis, or in a straight line. Place hands on the ground in front, near the thighs.

3 Inhale deeply and bend the upper body forwards. Let the hands slide up ahead on the ground, and continue to take deep breaths.

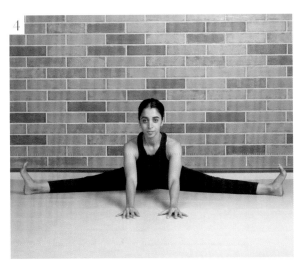

4 Slowly, walk the palms forwards while lowering the upper body bringing it as close to the floor as possible. The feet and legs should be stable and not move as the body bends at the hips.

5 In the final pose, the torso should be parallel to the ground and the arms should be stretched out in front. Hold this position for five breaths, then slowly return to the sitting position.

NAVASANA

This asana focuses on balance and core strength and engages the muscles in the abdomen. Its name translates to "boat pose" due to the appearance of the final posture. The practice of *Navasana* channels the steadiness and determination needed in a boat, fostering physical and mental resilience.

BENEFITS & CARE

Navasana stimulates kidneys, thyroid, and prostate glands, heightens full body awareness, improves digestion, while also working the core muscles and relieving tension. Those who are pregnant or have migraine, low blood pressure, spinal injuries, chronic neck pain, asthma, or heart issues should not attempt it.

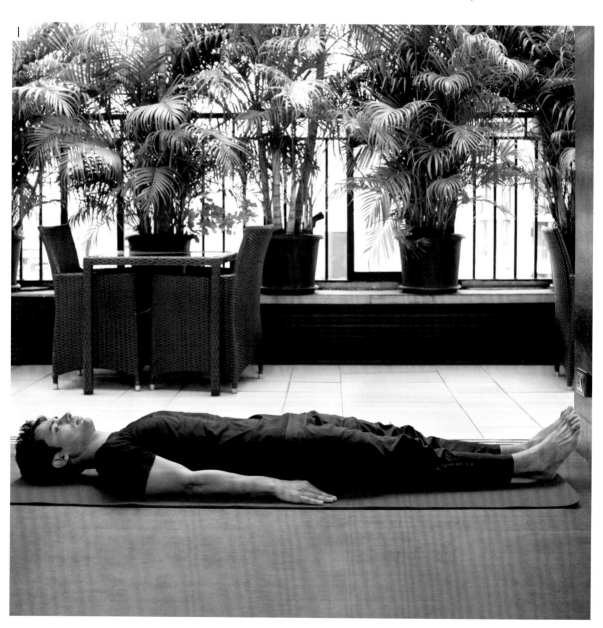

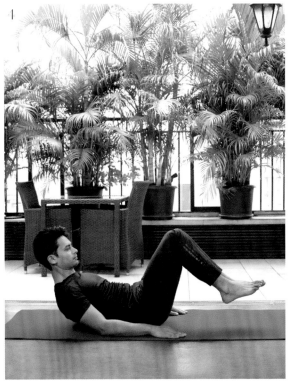

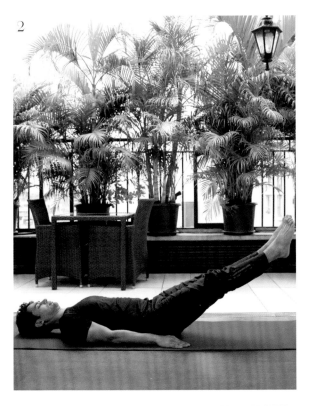

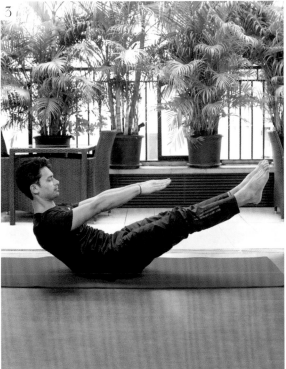

1. Lie on the ground facing upwards. Keep both feet together and arms straight on the side of the body. The palms should touch the ground.

2. Without lifting the arms, raise both feet off the ground. To start, the knees can be bent, but the shins must stay parallel to the ground.

3. Slowly lift the torso off the ground to create a "V" shape with the body. Keep the spine from rounding and hold the pose for five breaths.

4. If straightening the legs is difficult, start by keeping the knees folded. Raise the torso as much as possible and try to maintain balance.

UTPLUTHIH

Epitomizing balance and core strength, the *Utpluthih* is also called *Tolasana*, or "scale pose", due to how the body looks in the final posture. The arms symbolize balancing scales, and the asana fosters physical and mental equilibrium in yogic practice.

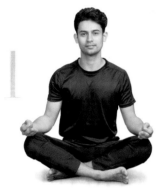

Sit cross-legged or in *Sukhasana* (see pp84–85). Place both the hands on the knees, palms facing upwards.

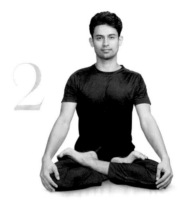

Lift the left leg and place on the right thigh, then lift the right leg and place on the left thigh. This is the "lotus pose".

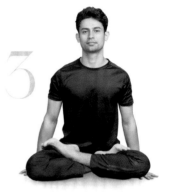

Place both palms firmly on the ground, outside the thighs, and tighten the abdominal muscles.

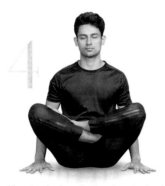

Elevate the legs by leaning the body backwards. Slowly raise the knees off the ground at a slight angle while still touching the ground with the hips.

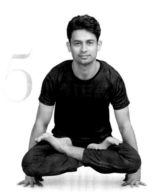

Distribute weight on the hands and raise the body upwards. Take care not to hurt the wrists and hold for five breaths, then return to the ground.

BHUJANGASANA

The final pose of the serpent-like *Bhujangasana* mimics a cobra with a raised hood. The reclining, back-bending asana is an important part of the *Surya Namaskar* (see pp180–185) and is good for toning and strengthening.

BENEFITS & CARE

Bhujangasana is great for strengthening the back, shoulders, and abdomen. It can be good for those with asthma as it expands the chest muscles and improves blood circulation. Pregnant practitioners, those suffering from hernia, ulcers, spondylitis, chronic back or spine problems, or those recovering from surgery should avoid the asana.

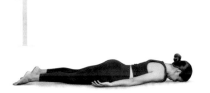

Assume the prone position on the ground. Keep both legs straight and toes together. The arms should be straight on either side of the body.

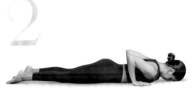

Slide both hands up towards the shoulder with the palms flat on the ground. Doing this will lift and bend the elbows.

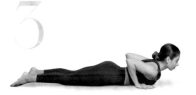

Elevate the upper body by exerting pressure on the palms to lift the torso, neck, and head from the ground.

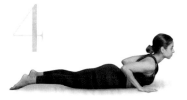

Keep the gaze in front. Put pressure on the hips, thighs, and shoulder blades to achieve a healthy arch of the back and neck.

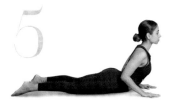

Continue to push upwards and raise the upper body as high as possible without locking the elbows. Hold for five breaths, then release.

IN FOCUS

Regular practice of the *Bhujangasana* tones the back and helps in the overall aim of weight loss. It helps organs such as the kidney and adrenal glands function better by compressing them during the practice.

JALANDHAR BANDHA

One of three main energy locks, or *bandha*, the *Jalandhar Bandha* involves the chin. It is practiced as part of advanced pranayama, or breathing practices, which activate different parts of the body to conduct deep breathing exercises.

BENEFITS & CARE

Jalandhar Bandha can stimulate the thyroid gland and regulate metabolism. It also promotes inner calm, breath retention, and concentration. Do not practice in case of breathing problems, heart conditions, or previous neck injury.

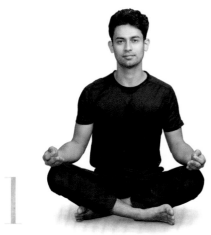

1 Sit in any cross-legged position, or in *Sukhasana* (see pp84–85). Rest both hands on the top of the knees.

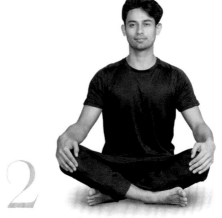

2 Inhale slowly and deeply while keeping the chest lifted. Hold the breath inside for as long as possible.

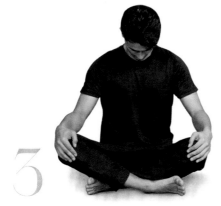

3 Tilt the head forwards and bring the chin to rest between the collarbones, on the jugular notch.

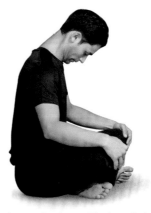

4 Focus all attention on the throat. The breath should be held until comfortably possible. Release when unable to hold longer and raise the chin.

ANULOM VILOM

Also known as "alternate nostril breathing", this core pranayama, or breathing technique, emphasizes cleansing and balancing the breath to calm the mind. As the name suggests, it involves inhaling and exhaling through one nostril at a time, or alternate nostrils, while holding the breath for a few moments in between.

BENEFITS & CARE

Anulom Vilom is great for respiratory, cardiovascular, and brain health. It improves focus, patience, and offers stress relief. Those who are pregnant, or suffer from chronic anxiety or hypertension should avoid it.

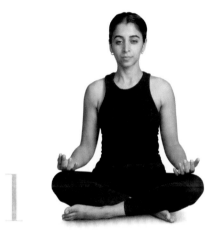

1
Sit in *Sukhasana* (see pp84–85) with a straight spine and neck. Close both eyes. Place both wrists on the knees and curve the middle and index fingers inwards.

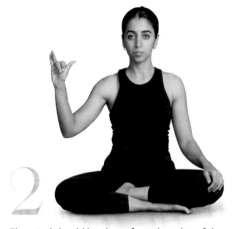

2
The mind should be clear of any thoughts of the past or future. Raise one hand and bring the index and middle fingers together as shown.

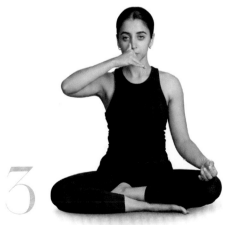

3
Cover the right nostril with the thumb and take a deep and slow breath from the left nostril until the lungs feel completely filled. Hold for five counts.

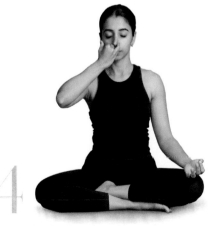

4
Release the thumb and use the ring finger to cover the left nostril. Exhale the breath through the right nostril. Repeat the asana alternating nostrils.

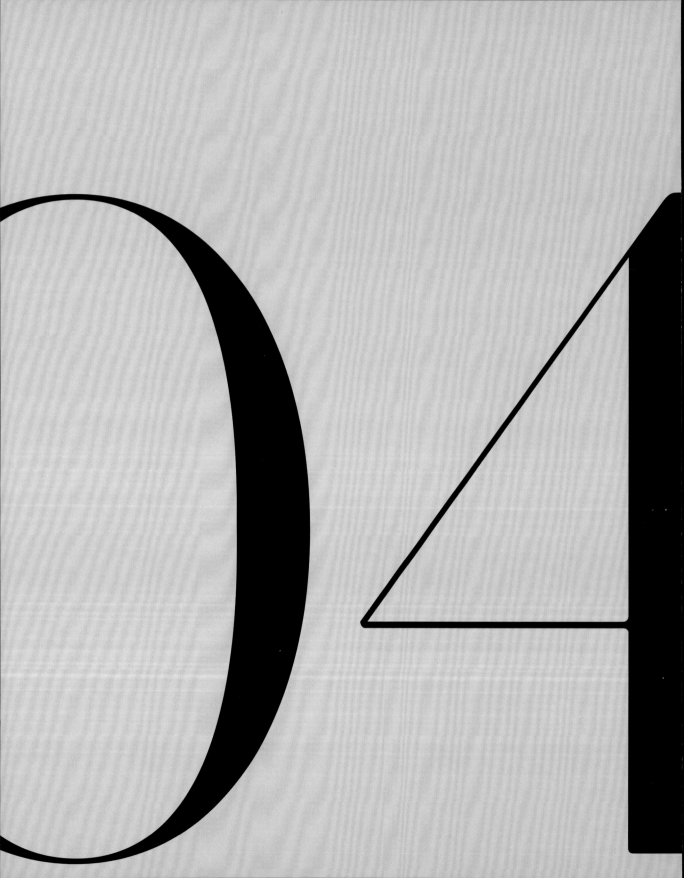

> "You need not worry or make yourself sleepless about the world; it will go on without you."
>
> SWAMI VIVEKANANDA, HINDU SPIRITUAL LEADER AND PROPONENT OF YOGA

WOMEN'S **HEALTH**

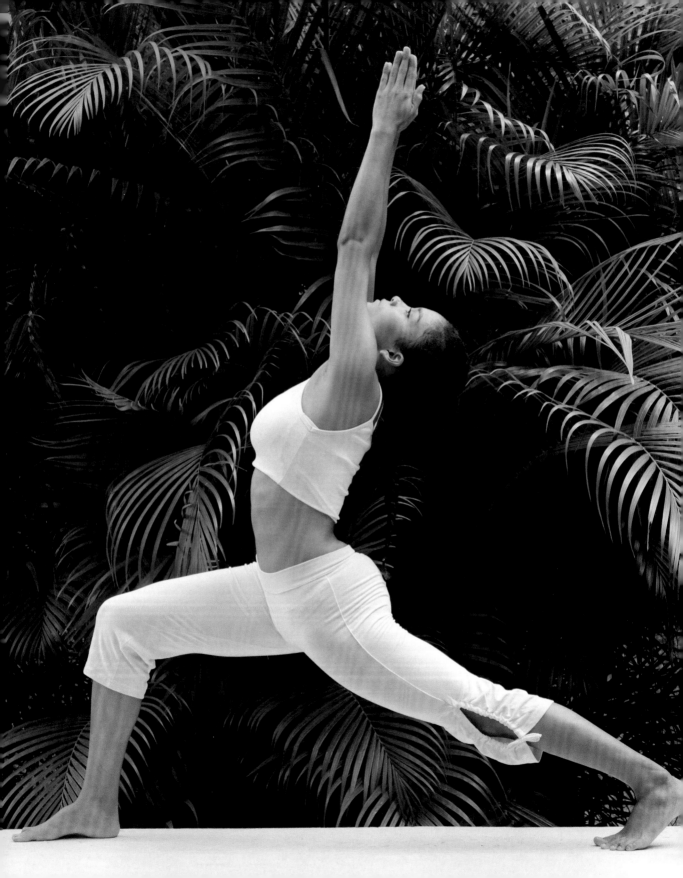

BALANCING HEALTH
WITH YOGA

Yoga is for everyone, whatever their age, level of fitness, gender, or lifestyle. It nurtures mental and physical wellbeing and has particular benefits for certain issues that affect women, including hormonal and reproductive health.

The gentle and effective practices of yoga bring about a balance in these systems of the body, including regulating menstrual cycles. Its stress-reducing techniques alleviate the impact of chronic stress on reproductive hormones, which fosters overall wellbeing.

Yoga is all about embracing and celebrating the unique journey of motherhood, and there are specific flows that are best suited for prenatal and postnatal care. From improved blood flow to reproductive organs, relief from menstrual discomfort, and reduced bloating to indirectly benefitting those trying to conceive, yoga helps promote women's health.

A critical benefit of yoga is that it can help to balance the hormones, which sit at the root of many medical issues. Hormonal imbalance can also be brought about as a result of external or internal factors. Often the roles that people play in their daily lives are so demanding that it creates situations of stress and imbalance. Yoga can help mitigate this and foster rejuvenation in such situations, whether the practitioner is a teenager or an adult woman.

A healthy lifestyle, which includes good food and sleeping habits as well as yoga and movement, enables progressive change. This encompasses all stages of one's life. For instance, prenatal yoga for expecting mothers is perhaps the most important disciplined inclusion they can make in their pregnancy routine. In such flows, yoga enables better mental health and fosters a deep connection between the mother and unborn child. It also has the potential to prepare the mother for a natural birth. Some simple, less-intensive exercises can be incorporated as early as two or three weeks after giving birth naturally (and about 12–16 weeks after a surgical birth).

Pranayama, or breathwork practices, such as *Anulom Vilom* (see p109) are the easiest to do from a pregnancy standpoint. Whereas, for maintaining hormonal health, asanas such as the *Bhujangasana* (see p107), the *Navasana* (see pp104–105), and the *Baddha Konasana* (see p125) are wonderful options. All it really takes is to carve out some time, just a few minutes each day and start small with something simple.

Every asana has its benefits and contraindications, and one should understand those carefully before engaging in routines. Listen to the body and don't push it into something harsh or painful from the first day. Only then will the rewards truly show.

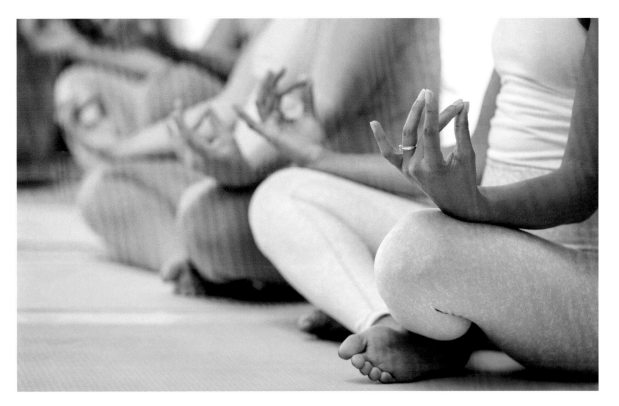

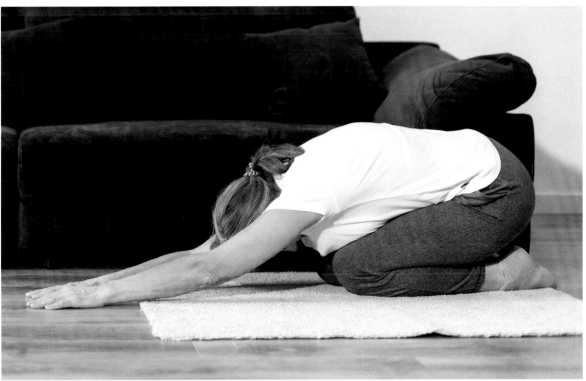

WOMEN'S HEALTH FLOW

From balancing hormones to managing menstrual pain, the benefits of yoga on the health of women is immense. This routine, starting with the *Sukhasana* (see p118) and ending with the *Dirga Pranayama* (see pp138–139) and *Dhyana* (see pp72–73), has been tailored to counter common health issues that impact women. Dedicated practice also benefits sleep pattern, enhances focus, and boosts metabolic function.

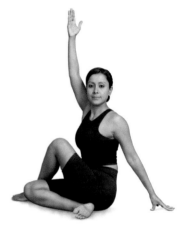

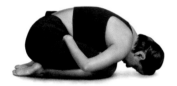

5 Mandukasana
Page 124

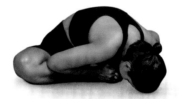

6 Baddha Konasana
Page 125

7 Ardha Matsyendrasana
Pages 126–127

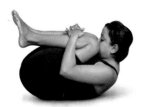

11 Pawanmuktasana
Page 131

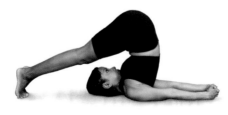

12 Halasana
Pages 132–133

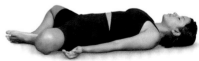

13 Supta Baddha Konasana
Pages 134–135

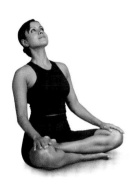

1 Sukhasana
Page 118

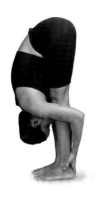

2 Uttanasana
Page 119

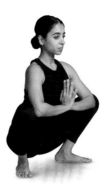

3 Malasana
Pages 120–121

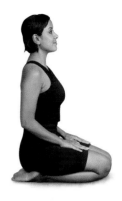

4 Vajrasana
Pages 122–123

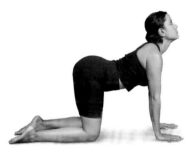

8 Bitilasana
Page 128

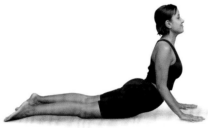

9 Bhujangasana
Page 129

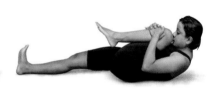

10 Ardha Pawan Muktasana
Page 130

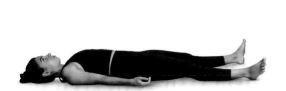

14 Savasana
Pages 136–137

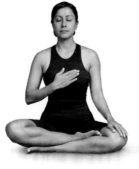

15 Dirga Pranayama
Pages 138–139

It is impactful to end every yoga flow or routine with a few moments of meditation. This is beneficial in bringing the mind and body back to a regulated sense of calm. Dedicated practice brings about an understanding of the self, and fosters steadiness of the mind and body, bringing it back to the present.

16 Dhyana
Pages 72–73

SUKHASANA

Many asanas are rooted in the *Sukhasana*, a simple yoga pose that is suitable for all levels of practitioners, including beginners. Regular practice of this asana positively impacts gut and digestive health, lengthens and straightens the spine, and promotes good posture.

BENEFITS & CARE

Sukhasana promotes relaxation and helps in meditation and breathing. It also eases lower back and knee pain. Avoid this asana in case of previous knee or hip injuries or in case of chronic knee pain.

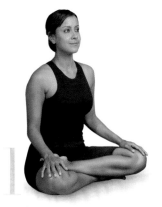

Start by sitting on a mat or ground with the spine straight and fold both legs at the knee. Bring the soles of the feet to rest under the opposite thighs.

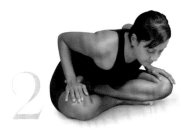

Keep the spine erect and place both hands on the knees. Feel the stretch in the lower back and start to lean down, facing forwards.

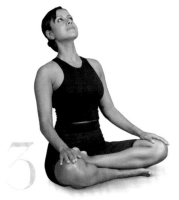

Sit back up and then slowly lean backwards. Ensure that the spine remains erect and the gaze is upwards.

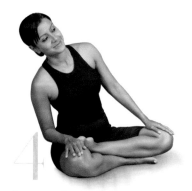

Return to the starting position. Begin to lean the body to the right. The right arm should rest on the thigh and the left should be taut.

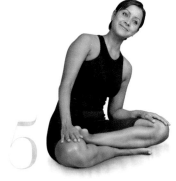

Repeat the movement on the other side, leaning the body towards the left. Hold each posture for a few breaths or until comfortable.

IN FOCUS

Practising *Sukhasana* asana as part of this flow regulates blood flow towards the upper body, especially to the abdominal organs. This aids in balanced and better functioning of those organs and helps manage health issues affecting the ovaries and the urinary tract. Many women also find that it also relieves severe headaches.

UTTANASANA

The "standing forward bend", or *Uttanasana*, encourages a sense of graceful surrender, calling on the practitioner to let go of tensions that are held by the body. The asana symbolizes the balance between making an effort and letting go, fostering physical and mental stillness.

BENEFITS & CARE

Uttanasana is good for improvement of posture and hip flexibility, and for relieving stiffness and tension in the back and neck. Avoid this asana in case of irregular blood pressure, glaucoma, osteoporosis, scoliosis, recent injuries, or surgeries.

IN FOCUS

Along with fostering relaxation, *Uttanasana*, in this flow, offers great relief from stomach pain during menstruation. Practising it regularly can aid in reducing premenstrual stress and relieving muscle stiffness.

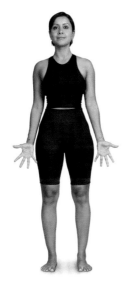

1

Stand straight with both feet parallel to one another and take a deep breath. Hands should be on the sides of the body with palms facing front.

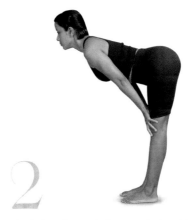

2

Slowly lean forwards, bowing the head first, while exhaling. Fold the lower trunk first, followed by the upper trunk. Let the hands rest on the thighs.

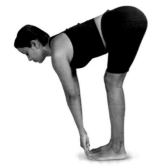

3

Continue to bend and reach down to touch the feet with the fingers, or place the palms on the ground. Keep the legs and arms straight and take a breath.

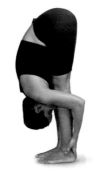

4

Continuing to breathe regularly, bring the forehead to the legs, or as low as is possible. Arms can hug the legs or touch the ground. Hold for five breaths.

MALASANA

Also known as the "Garland Pose", or the "Yogi Squat", *Malasana* is a grounding seated asana. In this pose, practitioners assume a deep squatting position, creating a shape reminiscent of a garland. It stretches the groin, hips, pelvis, and lower back areas, making it a great prenatal asana.

BENEFITS & CARE

Malasana increases metabolism, aids digestion, tones the abdomen, and keeps pelvic and hip joints healthy. Do not perform after a run, in case of hip or leg injuries, or with chronic back or knee pain.

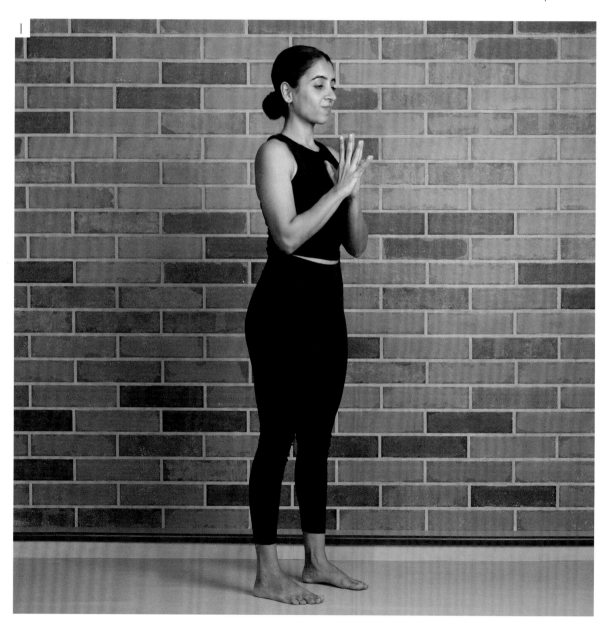

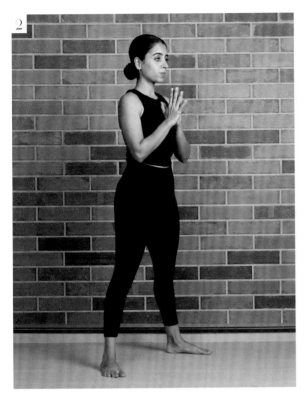

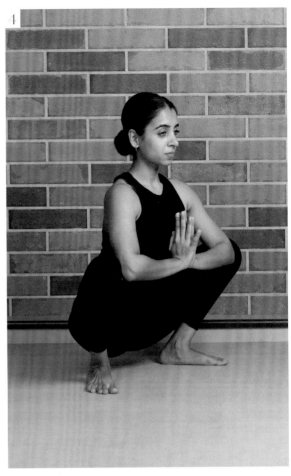

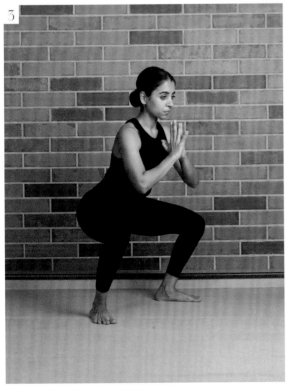

1 Stand straight with the feet parallel to one another. Join the hands with palms facing each other, and take regular breaths.

2 Spread the legs ensuring that the feet are about a foot apart. Keep the back straight and do not bend the knees.

3 Slowly lower the body down to a squat. Be sure to keep hands joined in front and that both heels are firmly on the ground.

4 Turn the feet outwards to maintain balance. Use the elbows to spread apart the upper legs to widen the squat. Hold this pose for five breaths.

VAJRASANA

In Sanskrit, *vajra* translates to either "thunderbolt", or "diamond", while asana means posture. The name symbolizes the strength and stability cultivated through this foundational seated pose that is often the starting point for many other asanas.

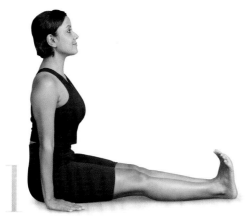

1 Start in a seated posture, both legs stretched in front, touching each other and toes pointing upwards. Keep the arms by either side with palms on the ground.

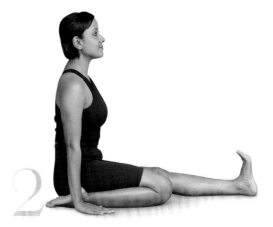

2 Fold one leg backwards, with the sole facing upwards. In case of any pain to the knee, use a folded blanket or cushion under the knees for support.

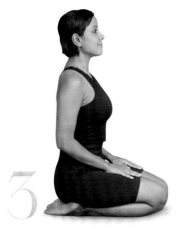

3 Fold the other leg and take a seat in the split space between the heels. Bring the big toes of both feet together. Keep the spine and neck straight, place both palms on the thighs, and hold the position for at least five breaths.

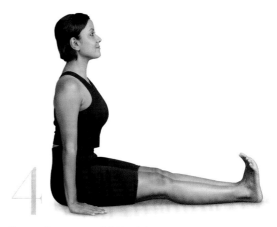

4 To exit the asana, unfold both legs, one at a time. Placing the palms on the ground for support, return to the starting position.

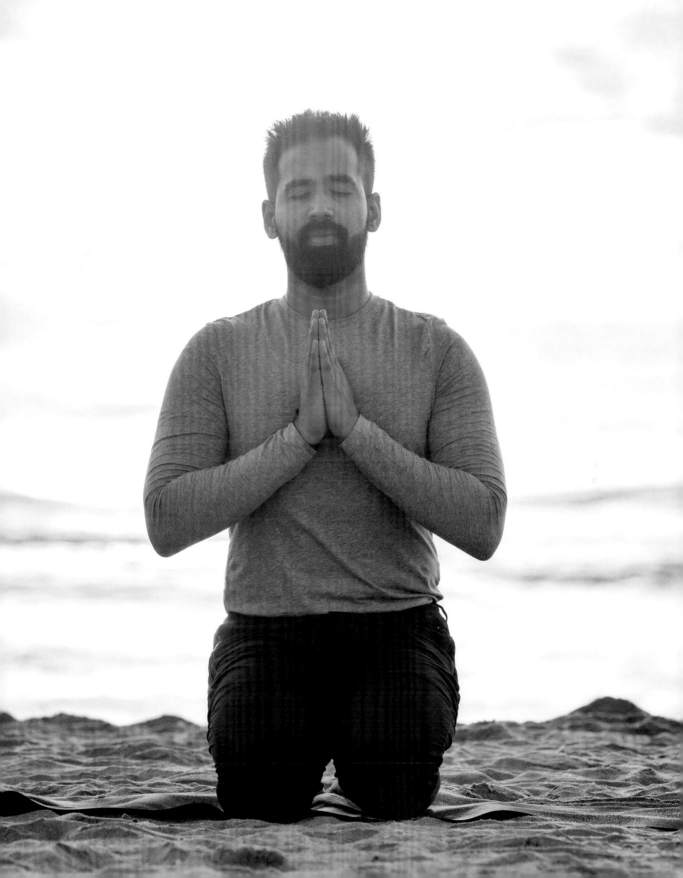

MANDUKASANA

In Sanskrit, *manduka* translates to "frog". *Mandukasana* is named for the frog-like appearance assumed in this posture, which also gives it its English name, the "frog pose". It is a unique and powerful yoga asana that embodies strength and flexibility. It is incorporated into yoga flows to enhance core strength and promote mental wellbeing.

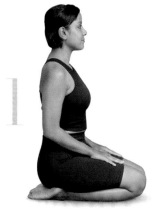

Assume the *Vajrasana* (see pp122–123). Both big toes should be tucked under the hips and touch each other.

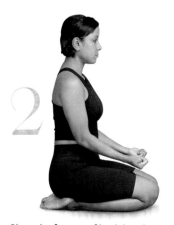

Close the fingers of both hands in a gentle fist with the thumbs at the base of the palm. This is the *Adi Mudra*.

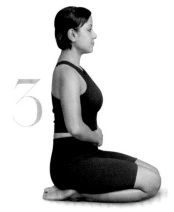

Place the fists in the *Adi Mudra* on either side of the navel and inhale deeply, then exhale completely.

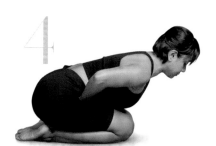

Slowly begin to lean forwards, keeping the back straight. Press the folded hands lightly into the abdomen while bending down.

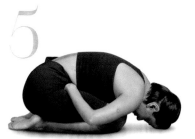

In the final pose, bend completely such that the crown of the head is touching the ground. Breathe deeply and hold this position for five breaths.

BADDHA KONASANA

The *Baddha Konasana* translates to "bound angle pose" and is also called the "butterfly pose" due to the position of the feet resembling the wings of a butterfly. This graceful asana lays emphasis on self reflection during its practice, and promotes the healthy functioning of the body.

BENEFITS & CARE

Baddha Konasana is known to aid in flexibility, improve blood circulation, and ease menstrual or menopausal discomfort. Do not attempt after knee, hip, or ankle surgery, or if suffering from injuries or arthritis.

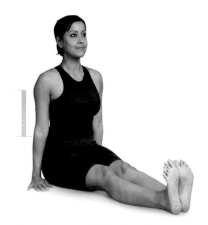

Sit on the ground with the back straight, arms on either side of the body, palms facing the ground, and legs stretched out in front.

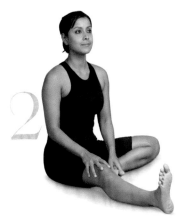

Fold the left leg and bring the sole of the foot close to the right knee. Hold in place with the left hand. The right hand should rest on the right knee.

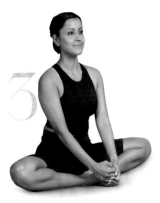

Draw the right leg to the same position by folding at the right knee. Let the soles of both feet touch and wrap both hands around the joined toes.

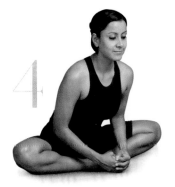

Lean down, keeping the back straight. The legs may feel as though they are unfolding like a book. Flap the knees up and down in the motion of wings.

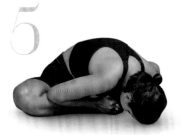

If comfortable, press the knees into the ground and lean down further until the crown of the head touches the ground in front. Hold this pose for five breaths.

ARDHA MATSYENDRASANA

The name of this pose translates to "half lord of the fishes", but it is also called the "sitting half spinal twist pose". It combines strength and spinal flexibility through a series of twisting and stretching movements. Expert practitioners perform this asana for the release of muscle tension that it fosters.

BENEFITS & CARE

Ardha Matsyendrasana burns fat, opens the chest, improves oxygen circulation, and increases elasticity of the spine. Do not try if menstruating, pregnant, or suffering from spinal injuries, peptic ulcers, or a hernia.

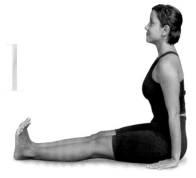

Sit with legs stretched out in front. Keep the back straight, join the feet, and bring both hands to either side of the body.

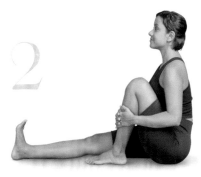

Bend the left leg at the knee. Use the hands to pull the foot closer to the body so the heel is close to the thigh.

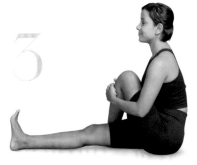

Lift the left foot and bring it to the outside of the right thigh. The hands can be wrapped around the knee for this.

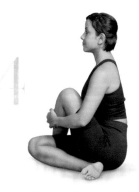

Slowly fold the right leg such that the heel of the foot touches the glutes on the left side.

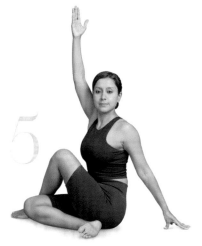

Let the left arm rest on the ground behind the body for support. Raise the right hand, and rotate the head, trunk, and arm slowly towards the left.

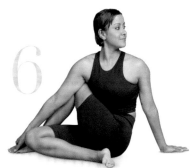

Facing the back, bring the right hand to hold the left big toe. The right elbow should touch the outside of the left knee. Hold for five breaths, repeat on the other side.

"It is the power to focus the consciousness on a given spot, and hold it there. Attention is the first and indispensable step in all knowledge."

PATANJALI, AUTHOR, MYSTIC, AND PHILOSOPHER, c.401–500 CE

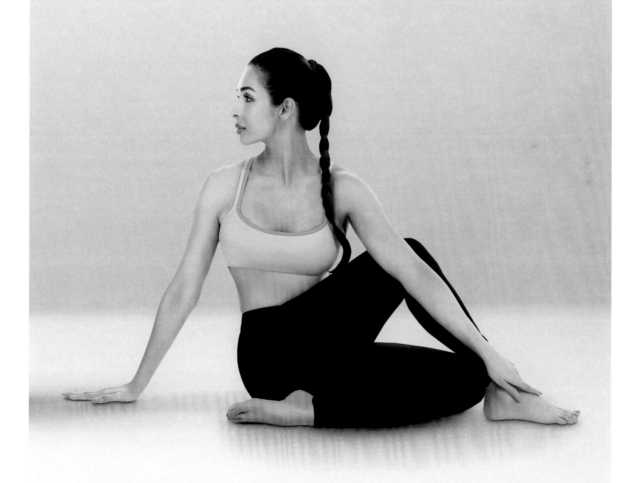

BITILASANA

Bitilasana, or "cow pose", is a gentle and easy asana that focuses on the co-ordination of breath and flexibility of the spine. This asana is frequently used as a transition pose or as part of a warm-up routine before more intensive yoga sessions.

BENEFITS & CARE

Bitilasana is great for spinal flexibility, relieving shoulder, neck, and back tension, engaging core muscles, strengthening joints in the wrists, hips, and knees. It encourages better sleep and is a good addition to prenatal and postnatal flows. It should be avoided in case of irregular blood pressure, arthritis, spondylitis, or other injuries to the shoulders, wrists, neck, hip, knee or back.

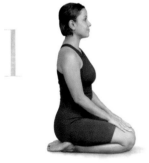

Begin by assuming the *Vajrasana* posture (see pp122–123). Keep the spine erect and look straight ahead.

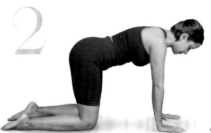

Place both hands firmly on the ground in front and lean forwards. The arms should be shoulder-distance apart.

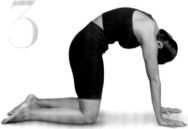

Push into the ground using the hands. Expand the collarbones with a deep inhalation. Elevate the chest and chin, and drop the belly to arch the back.

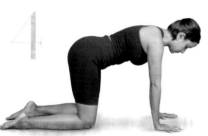

Slowly return to a neutral position with the spine straightened. This is known as the table-top position. Keep the head facing downwards in this pose.

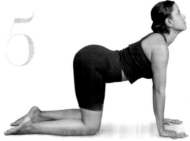

To achieve the final pose, lower the spine in a reverse-arch. Exert pressure on the ground with the hands and look upwards as the body stretches. Repeat this five times.

BHUJANGASANA

One of the most accessible yoga poses, "cobra pose" or *Bhujangasana* is taught to all levels of practitioners as a back bending warm-up pose before more rigorous asanas. However, its simple steps make it a great quick pose to practice on its own every day as well.

BENEFITS & CARE

Apart from stretching the ankle dorsiflexors, hip flexors, abdominals, biceps, cervical flexors, and pectoralis muscles, *Bhujangasana* can improve sleep and reduce inflammation. Do not attempt if pregnant, in case of wrist or rib fracture, spondylitis, recent surgeries, or experiencing asthma.

IN FOCUS

When included into a yoga flow focused on women's health, this asana impacts the ovaries and the uterus. It also has a significant impact on the organs in the abdomen area. Some yoga teachers recommend it for treating disorders such as leucorrhoea, painful menstrual cycles, and amenorrhoea.

1

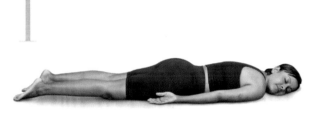

Lie down in the prone position. Keep the legs straight and the toes touching the ground. Both hands should be on either side of the body, palms facing upwards.

2

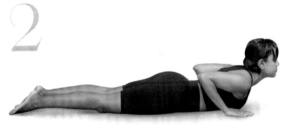

Bring the hands up towards the shoulders. Bend at the elbows and lay both palms firmly on the ground. The head should lift up slowly, but the gaze should remain in front.

3

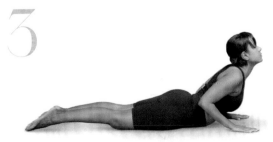

Start raising the upper body, lifting the chest and neck off the ground. To do this, push up by pressing the palms into the ground and look upwards.

4

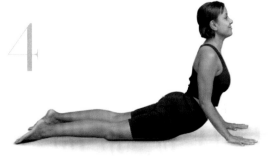

Exert gentle pressure on the hips, thighs, and shoulder blades, and raise the body higher until an arch is created. Hold for five breaths, then release.

ARDHA PAWAN MUKTASANA

The "half wind-relieving pose", or *Ardha Pawan Muktasana*, is a simple-yet-effective, restorative asana that releases tension in the lower back, and unwanted gas from the abdominal region. It prepares the spine and back muscles for intense supine poses.

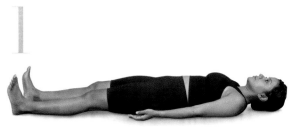

1. Lie on the back with the legs slightly apart, hands relaxed on the sides, and the lower back resting or touching the ground.

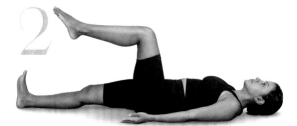

2. Exhale and employ the muscles in the core to lift the left leg to a 60-degree angle. Bend the left knee but be sure to keep the right leg extended.

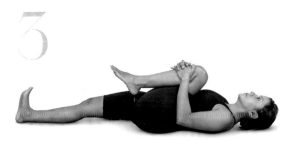

3. Wrap both hands around the shin and press the left thigh into the left side of the chest. Do not hold the breath, or any tension or gas in.

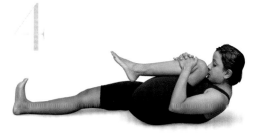

4. Hug the leg tighter, lift the neck, and bend down to touch the nose or the forehead to the knee. Hold this for as long as comfortable, release, and then repeat with the right leg.

PAWANMUKTASANA

An effective asana for the healthy functioning of the digestive system, the *Pawanmuktasana* or the "wind-relieving pose" is a variation of the *Ardha Pawan Muktasana* (see p130). This restorative yoga pose is easy to perform and can be practised every morning.

BENEFITS & CARE

Pawanmuktasana massages the pelvic muscles and reproductive organs and is beneficial for menstrual disorders. It tones the abdomen, thighs and glutes, releases trapped gases, and improves blood circulation. Avoid it in case of heart ailments, high blood pressure, pregnancy, injuries, haemorrhoids, or slipped disc.

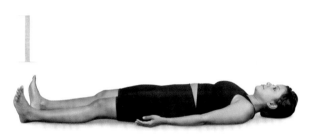

1

Lie on the back with legs slightly apart, hands relaxed on the sides, and the lower back resting or touching the ground.

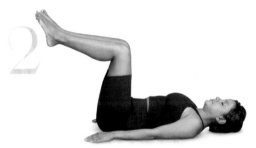

2

On an exhalation, engage the core muscles to lift both legs off the ground. Raise to a 60-degree angle at the knee and hold.

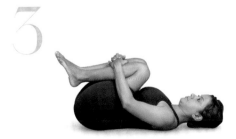

3

Bring the calves of both feet to the thighs. Bring the knees as close to the chest as possible and wrap arms around the knees to hug them to the chest.

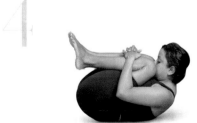

4

Raise the neck to touch the forehead or the nose to the knee. Hold for as long as possible. In case of any discomfort, do not raise the head, but hold pose as shown in step 3.

HALASANA

Halasana, commonly known as "plough pose", is a graceful and invigorating inversion pose. In Sanskrit, *hala* means "plough", and the asana highlights this distinctive shape in the final pose. When practised mindfully, this rejuvenating posture promotes a sense of calm and relaxation.

BENEFITS & CARE

Halasana is great for spinal flexibility, loosening tightness in the hamstrings, regulating blood sugar, easing discomfort from haemorrhoids, and stimulating the thyroid gland. Avoid it in case of cervical pain, abdominal injury, hernia, or if pregnant.

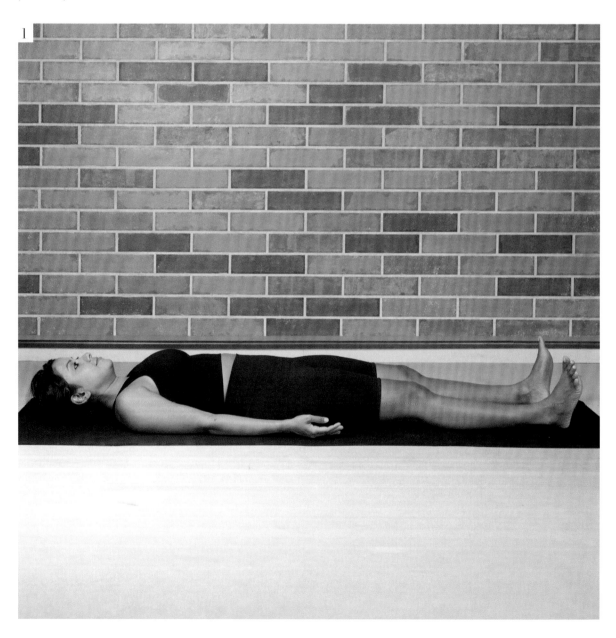

1

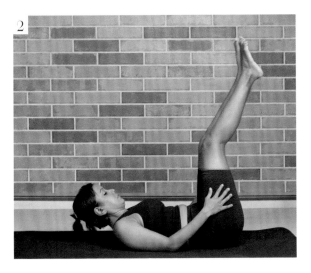

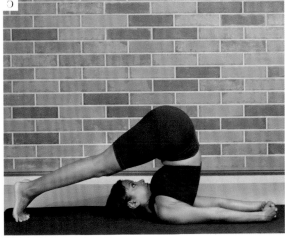

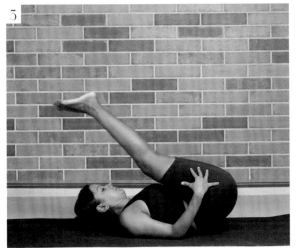

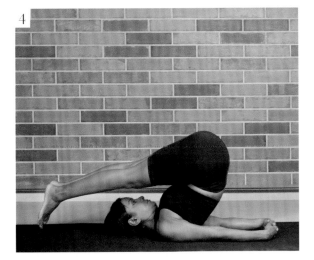

1   Lie on the back and take a few calm and deep breaths. In this position, the legs should be joined and hands on either side of the body with palms facing up.

2   Raise both legs off the ground until perpendicular by engaging the core muscles. Maintain a compact and straight stance. The hands can rest on the thighs.

3   Slowly raise the glutes and hips off the ground. Roll the spine until the feet lift up and behind the head. The legs should remain straight.

4   Pushing the legs backwards by raising the back. Spine should be straight and hands back in the resting position, fingers joined. The toes should touch the ground.

5   Continue pushing until the final posture, where the spine is parallel to the ground, is achieved. Hold for five breaths. If needed, use the hands on the back for support.

IN FOCUS

Halasana has an effect on the thyroid and parathyroid glands which are situated in the neck region. Teachers also recommend it for urinary disorders, menstrual issues, haemorrhoids, and hernia.

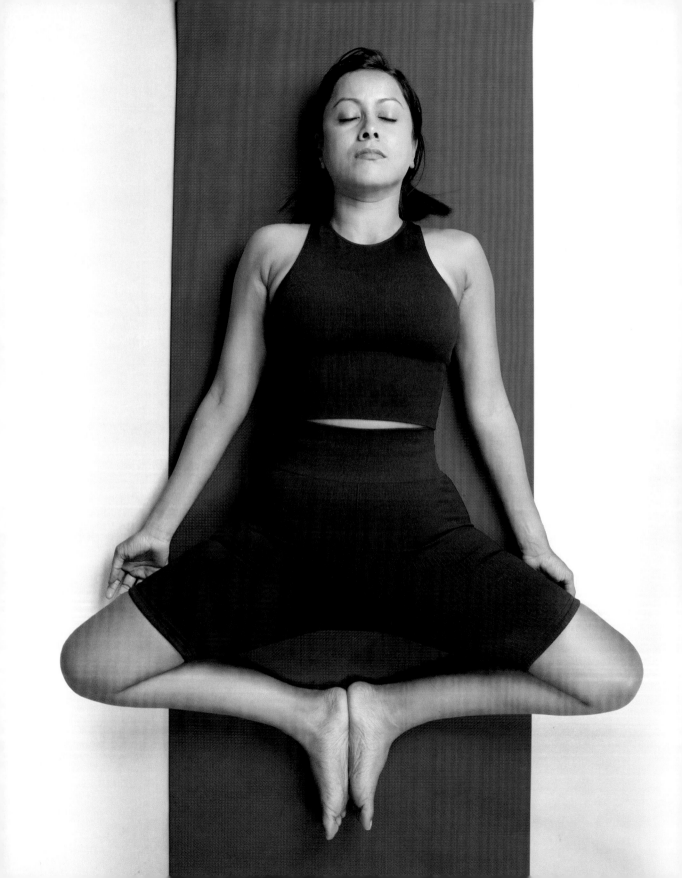

SUPTA BADDHA KONASANA

The "reclining bound angle pose", "goddess pose", or *Supta Baddha Konasana*, is a deeply restorative and heart-opening asana. It is often practised as a restorative pose to bring about a sense of inner calm and balance.

BENEFITS & CARE

Supta Baddha Konasana activates the ovaries, benefits the kidneys, improves blood circulation, induces sleep, and is great for alleviating tension. Avoid in case of hip or knee injury, or hip or back pain. If pregnant, perform only under expert supervision.

1

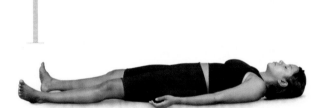

Lie on the back and take a few deep breaths. Keep the arms on either sides of the body, with the palms facing up, and the legs relaxed and slightly apart.

2

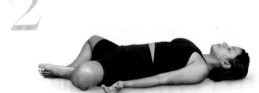

Extend the knees to the sides and bring the soles together. The legs should be as in the *Baddha Konasana* (see p125). Rest the arms and breathe normally. Hold the pose for a few minutes, allowing gravity to deepen the stretch. At the end of the asana, remember to move into *Savasana* (see pp66–67) to calm the mind, before getting into breathwork.

> "
> Chalk out a programme of life. Draw your spiritual routine. Stick to it systematically and regularly. Apply yourself diligently. Waste not even a single precious minute. Life is short. Time is fleeting. That "tomorrow" will never come. Now or never.
>
> SWAMI SIVANANDA SARASWATI, NOTED YOGA GURU AND PHYSICIAN
> "

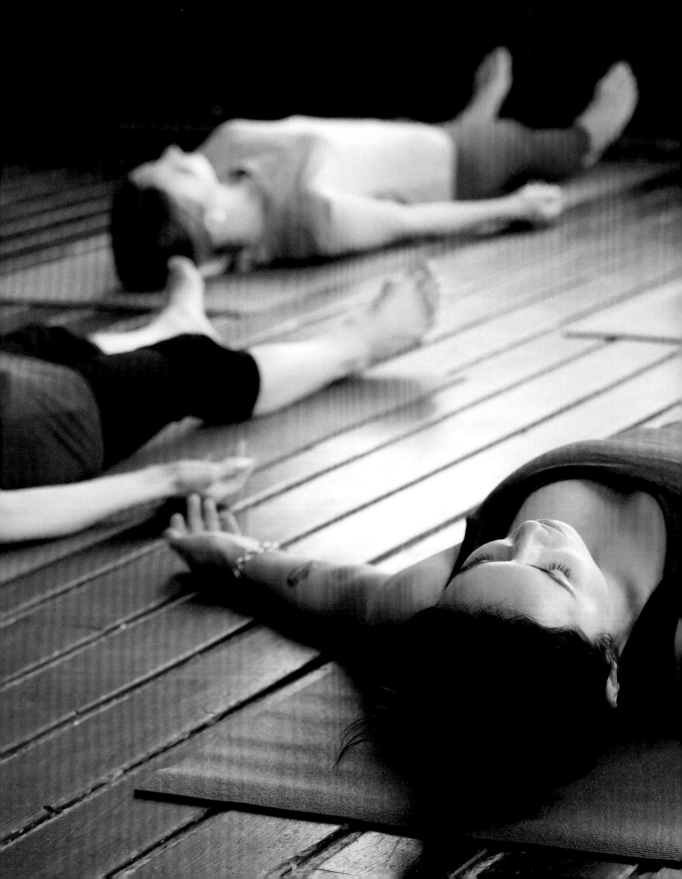

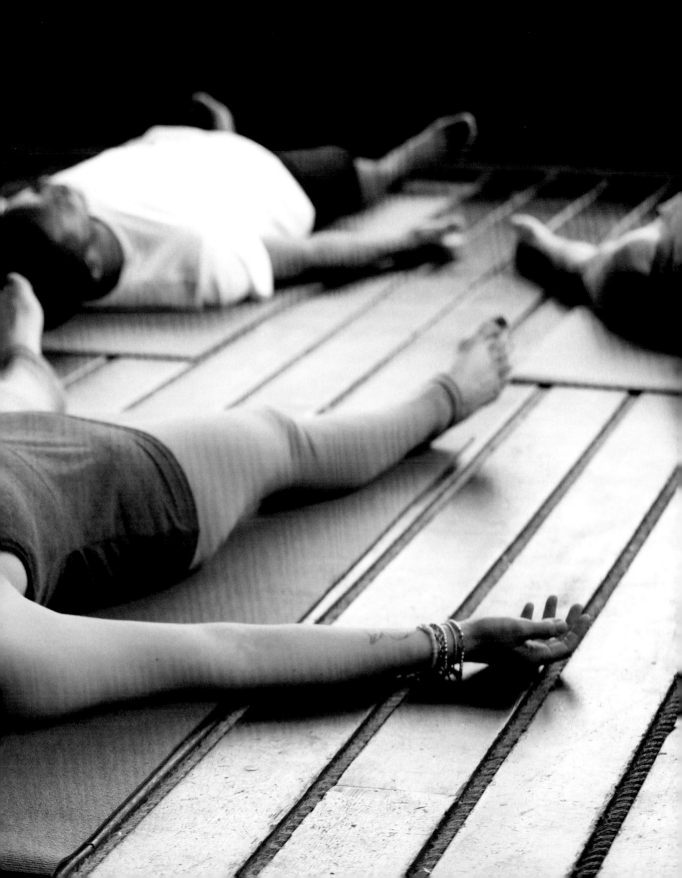

DIRGA PRANAYAMA

"Three-part breath" is a grounding breathing exercise that is often recommended to beginners and experts alike. It works as a great transitional exercise at the beginning or ending of a routine as it helps to attune the practitioner back to the present.

BENEFITS & CARE

Dirga Pranayama regulates breath, brings about a heightened awareness of the self, and reduces anxiety. Anyone can do the asana but don't hold the breath in if pregnant or having heart, lung, eye, ear problems, or high blood pressure.

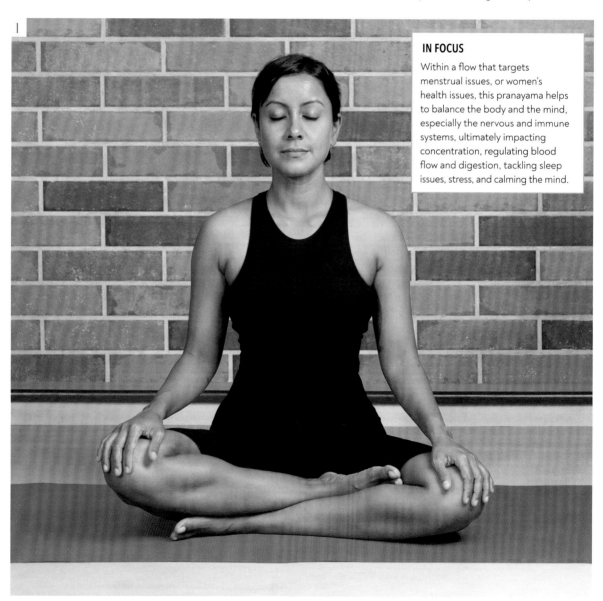

IN FOCUS

Within a flow that targets menstrual issues, or women's health issues, this pranayama helps to balance the body and the mind, especially the nervous and immune systems, ultimately impacting concentration, regulating blood flow and digestion, tackling sleep issues, stress, and calming the mind.

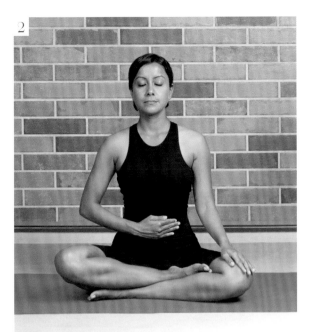

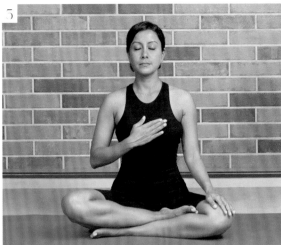

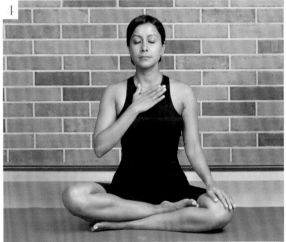

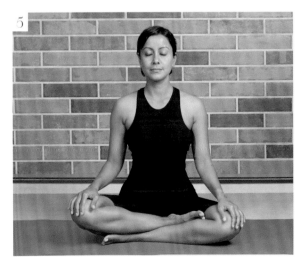

1   Sit with legs crossed and both eyes closed. Get comfortable and start by noticing the breath while inhaling and exhaling naturally. If distracted, bring the focus back to the way the breath feels.

2   Take long and deep breaths and let the air fill the belly with each inhalation. Place a hand on the belly to feel the inflation. Repeat for five breaths.

3   Let the air expand the lungs, spreading the ribcage apart as it does. Move the hand to the chest to feel this and repeat for five breaths.

4   Exhale and let the air out of the lungs first, then the belly. Contract the navel inwards. After five breaths, repeat step 3 but feel the air fill the upper chest with a hand placed on the heart.

5   When exhaling, let the breath exit the chest first, then the lungs, and then the belly, once again contracting the navel inwards. Repeat for 10 breaths.

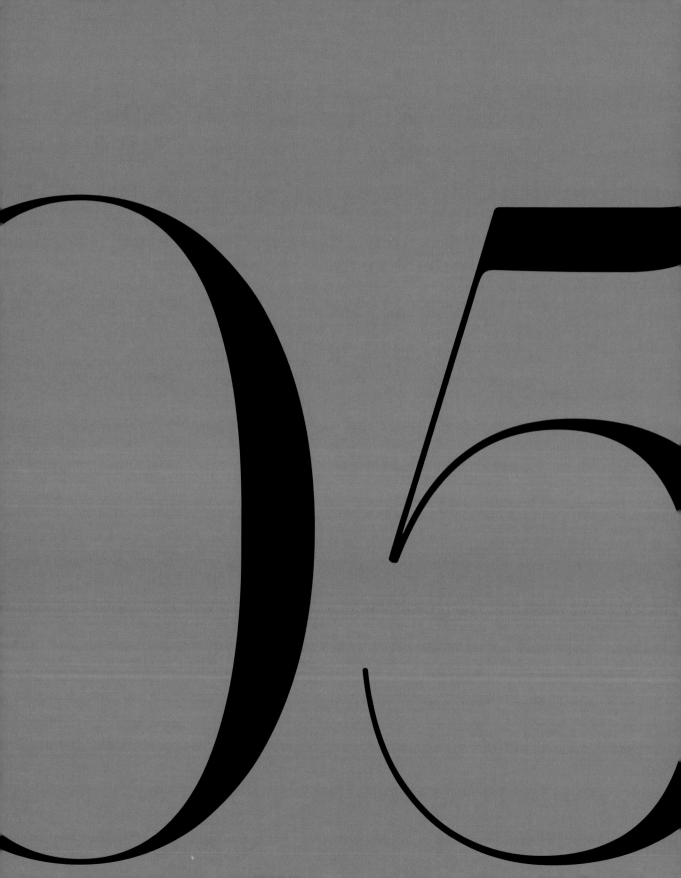

SUPERHUMAN

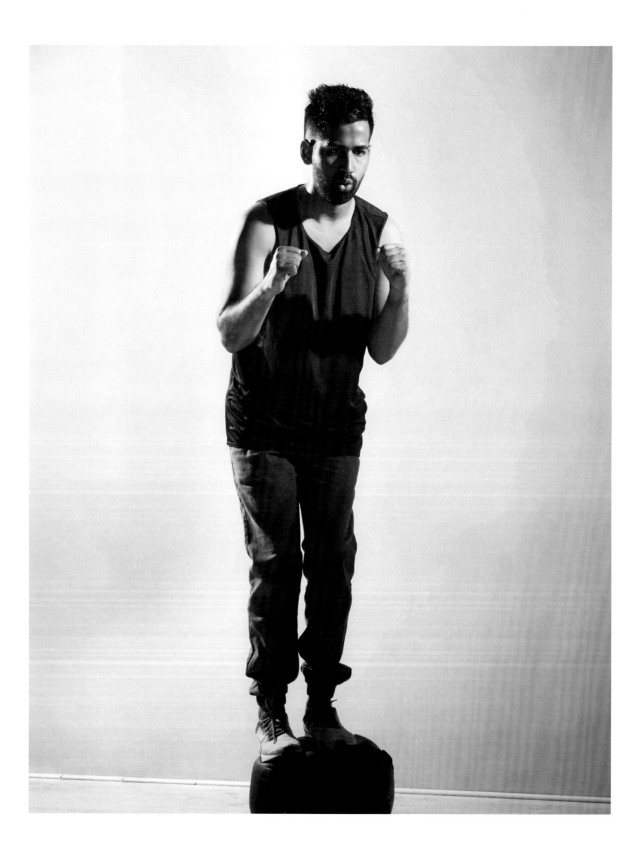

GENERAL FITNESS
THROUGH YOGA

The practice of yoga is where strength finds serenity, flexibility meets focus, and champions are born anew. I always say that in yoga, like in football or soccer, it's not about the goals, but about the beautiful game that takes place. Dedicated practice can help unlock the full potential of the body and the mind. On one hand, yoga improves flexibility, strength, and balance, which can make one feel more capable and agile. On another, it gives the practitioner mental clarity and a great boost of energy, ready to take on challenges.

Though it does not grant superpowers, yoga builds the tools needed to tap into one's innate potential, contributes to a longer, healthier life, making one feel superhuman in terms of vitality and wellbeing, and incorporates more resilience in one's daily life. Unfortunately, yoga is often overlooked as an option when one begins the fitness journey, with the practitioner opting for more seemingly high-intensity exercises.

I can't begin to stress the importance of yoga in one's overall wellbeing. One can start this journey at any stage of one's life, even those who are already on the path to fitness.

In fact, yoga helps build strength to help with other forms of exercise. To lift weights, one must have a strong back, and asanas such as the *Bitilasana* (see p128), can help in building those muscles. Similarly, there are asanas that can help strengthen the knee, while some pranayamas are a great way to clear the respiratory system, improve lung function, and aid in recovery post-COVID-19 or even the flu.

Experienced practitioners and teachers can tailor routines that target all parts of the body. They can also build awareness about the body and the self – the latter comes through the practice of *Dhyana* (see pp72–73) and breathwork. In any exercise routine, warming up and cooling down are of utmost importance. Yoga is no different. Adding meditative relaxation to the cool-down routine will alleviate anxiety and allow the tensions we store in our muscles to dissipate. The most important change that yoga brings is the vitality and energy to get through a day. It clears doubts, eliminates worries, and rejuvenates the body – it is also one of

the simplest ways to incorporate exercise into one's life. *Anulom Vilom* (see p109), for example, has no contraindications associated with it. A 9-year-old can do it just as well as a 90-year-old. All one needs is a mat and a will to try.

Over the past many years, I have seen my body change, but I have been the happiest when I am engaging in yoga every day. It helps me sleep, and better understand and respect my body and its capabilities. The yoga asanas and pranayamas in this chapter follow the simple four-fold rule – warm up, perform asanas, cool down, and commit to pranayamas and meditation. When practised with commitment and authenticity, yoga can solve most problems that plague our lives today.

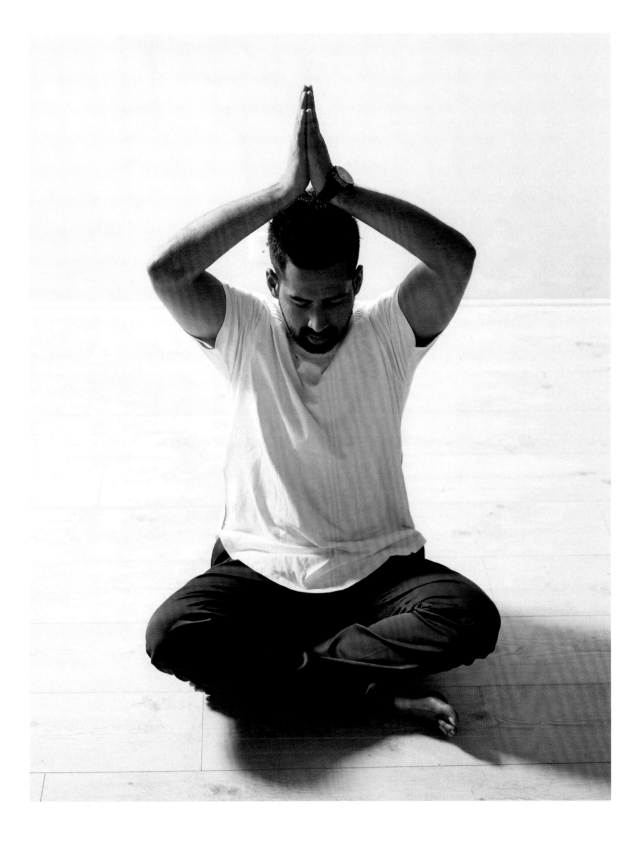

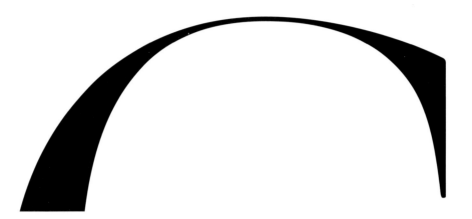

CONNECT with your surroundings for five minutes every day. Experience nature, count your blessings, and thank the universe for all the little things that you have. Inculcating gratitude is a way for us to find love for the community we inhabit, the world around us, and in turn, ourselves. Spending a few simple moments will strengthen your sense of empathy and compassion, which will help you embrace and celebrate the interconnectedness of all beings. This connection is central to any yogic practice. Connect regularly in this way for a week, and you will see the difference and find your own path towards a harmonious existence.

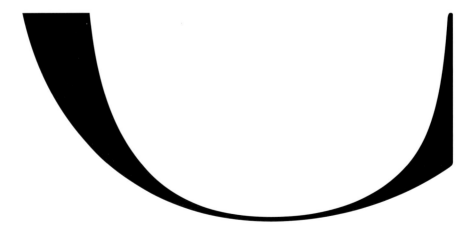

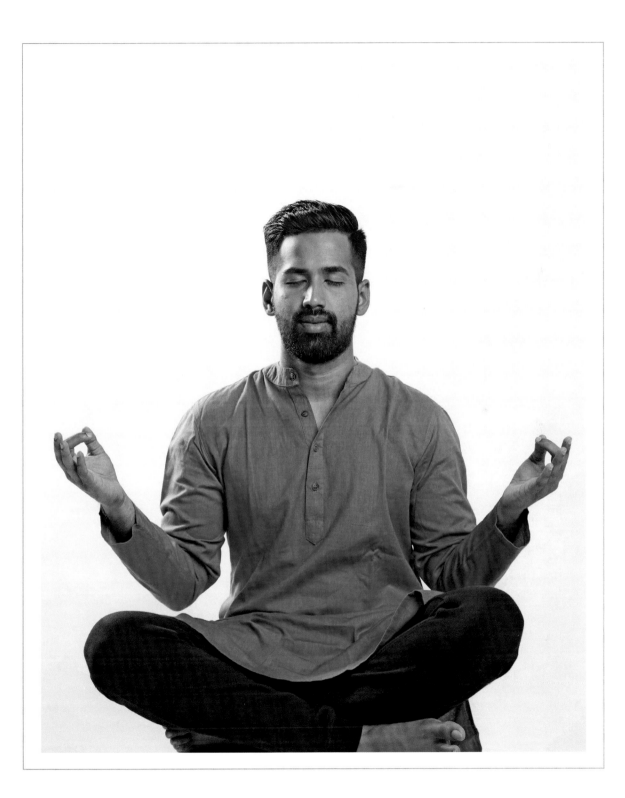

SUPERHUMAN FLOW

Yoga is a transformational combination of asanas or postures, *dhyana* or meditation, and pranayama or breathwork. Together, these components help build everything from muscle strength, flexibility, balance, and stamina to mindfulness, calmness, and focus. This sequence, from *Adham Pranayama* (see p150) to *Sitkari* (see pp174–175) and *Dhyana* (see pp72–73) is a complete flow best suited for overall health and fitness.

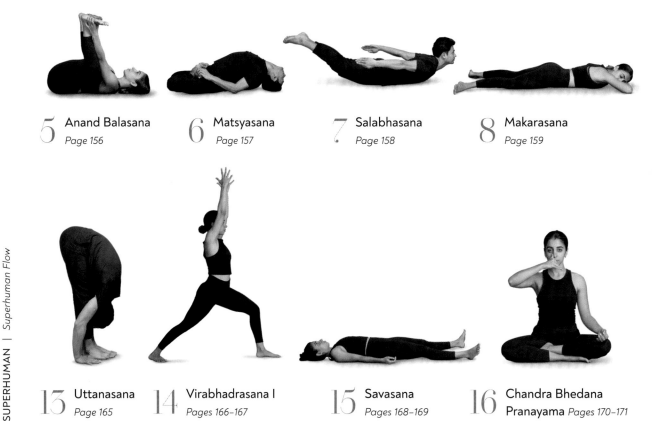

5 **Anand Balasana**
Page 156

6 **Matsyasana**
Page 157

7 **Salabhasana**
Page 158

8 **Makarasana**
Page 159

13 **Uttanasana**
Page 165

14 **Virabhadrasana I**
Pages 166–167

15 **Savasana**
Pages 168–169

16 **Chandra Bhedana Pranayama** *Pages 170–171*

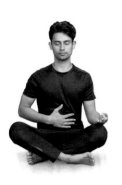

1 Adham Pranayama
Page 150

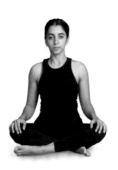

2 Sukhasana
Page 151

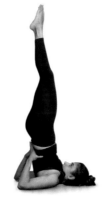

3 Sarvangasana
Pages 152–153

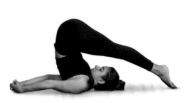

4 Halasana
Pages 154–155

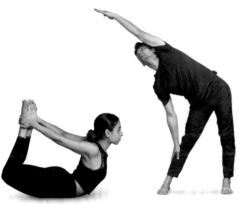

9 Dhanurasana
Pages 160–161

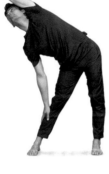

10 Konasana
Page 162

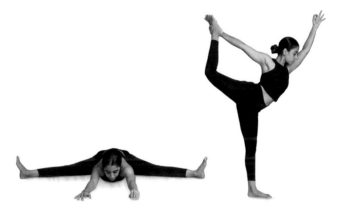

11 Upavistha Konasana
Page 163

12 Natarajasana
Page 164

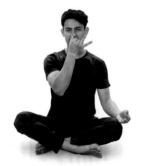

17 Surya Bhedana Pranayama
Pages 172–173

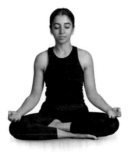

18 Sitkari
Pages 174–175

End every yoga flow, or routine, with a few moments of meditation. This will bring the mind and body back to a regulated sense of calm and foster equilibrium. Dedicated practice brings about an understanding of the self, including fostering a better relationship with food, the body, and exercise.

19 Dhyana
Pages 72–73

ADHAM PRANAYAMA

BENEFITS & CARE

Adham pranayama strengthens abdominal muscles, aides in digestion, and relaxes the body. Only the abdomen should rise and fall and the chest should not be inflated.

Also known as "diaphragmatic breathing" or "belly breathing", this seated asana is a powerful and effective technique that focuses on harnessing the full capacity of the breath. It calms and soothes both the body and the mind.

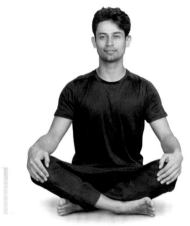

1. Sit on the floor with the spine straight. If the back needs support, sit on a chair with both feet placed flat on the ground.

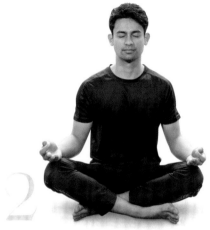

2. Close the eyes and take several long, deep breaths. Focus on the breath while allowing the body to relax. The face, neck, and shoulders should not be tense.

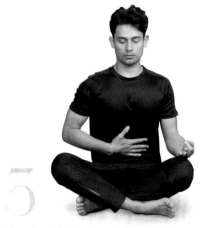

3. Place the right hand on the stomach. Take a deep breath and hold until the stomach pushes against the palm. With a gentle exhale, feel the stomach move towards the spine.

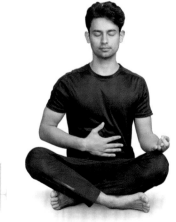

4. Strive to breathe deeply and slowly, allowing the stomach to move gently. Attempt to keep the chest as still as possible. Continue deep breathing for a few minutes.

SUKHASANA

Practised in preparation for meditation and breathing exercises, Sukhasana involves adopting a simple cross-legged position. This asana helps provide a firm and stable base for the body, and keeps the energy centred.

BENEFITS & CARE

Sukhasana helps in meditation and breathing and promotes relaxation. It also eases lower back and knee pain. Avoid this asana in case of previous knee or hip injuries, or chronic knee or back pain.

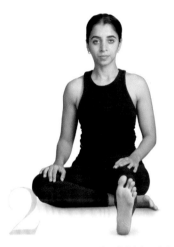

1 Sit with both legs stretched in front. The neck and back should remain straight at all times.

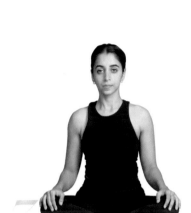

2 Keep the spine straight, fold the right leg at the knee, and bring the sole of the foot to rest under the other thigh.

3 Repeat the same movement with the other leg and adjust the seating position so as to feel minimal pressure on both ankles.

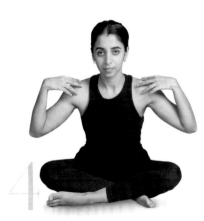

4 Place the palms on the shoulders and gently slide the shoulder back to its original resting position. Keep the head raised and the crown facing up.

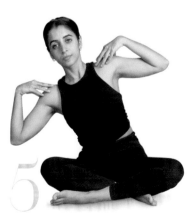

5 Maintaining the position of the head, move side to side. Breathe normally. Repeat as many times as needed to feel "loose" enough to begin other asanas.

IN FOCUS

Sukhasana is a great tool for a flow focused on general fitness. It builds overall stability and mobility, strengthens the back muscles and the lower half of the body, and improves the posture as it lengthens the spines.

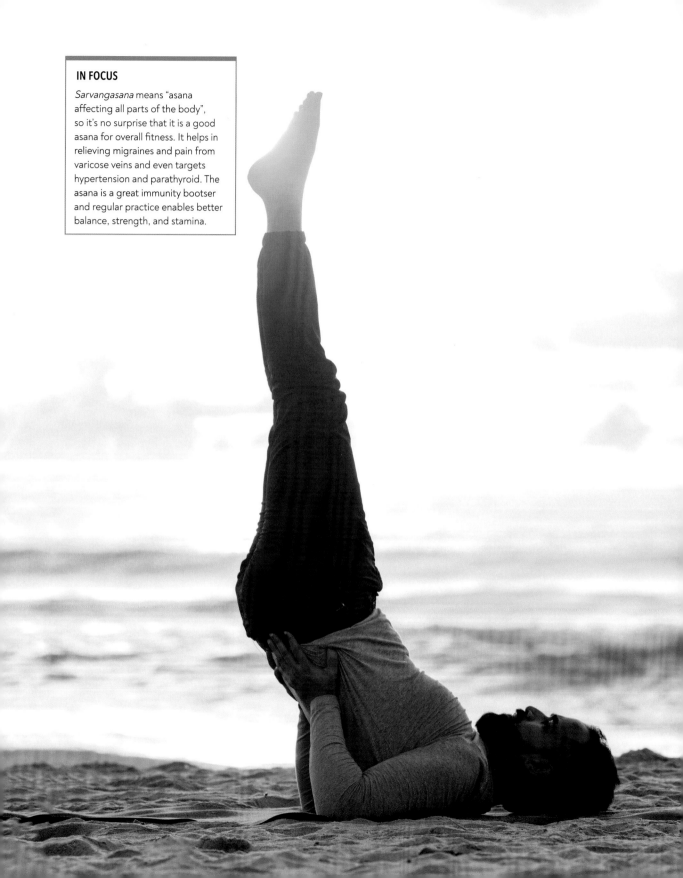

IN FOCUS

Sarvangasana means "asana affecting all parts of the body", so it's no surprise that it is a good asana for overall fitness. It helps in relieving migraines and pain from varicose veins and even targets hypertension and parathyroid. The asana is a great immunity bootser and regular practice enables better balance, strength, and stamina.

SARVANGASANA

A foundational yoga pose that promotes balance and harmony, the *Sarvangasana* works on the full body. Also called the "shoulder stand", this inverted posture may seem daunting at first, but with some practice, it can be quite easy to perform.

BENEFITS & CARE

This asana helps relieve headaches and issues with the ear, nose, and throat. It is great for posture and building upper back strength. Avoid it in case of any injuries to the back or spine, or if suffering from spondylitis or other chronic pain conditions.

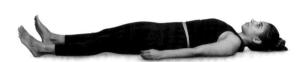

Lie on the back with feet slightly apart and both arms on either side of the body.

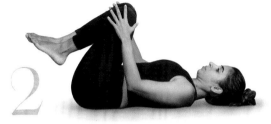

2 Slowly raise the legs and the hips off the ground, bending the legs at the knee. If needed, support them with hands placed on either side.

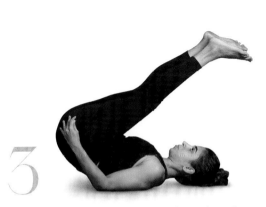

3 Use the hands to support the hips and straighten the legs, extending them to the back.

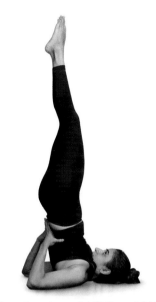

4 Now, straighten the spine and shift the weight from the shoulders to the arms, moving both hands to the back for support. Hold for 30 seconds or more.

HALASANA

When it comes to overall fitness, asanas, such as the *Halasana*, which target different areas of the body, are important to include in a sequence. It is usually considered a finishing asana practiced at the end of different routines due to the relaxation is fosters.

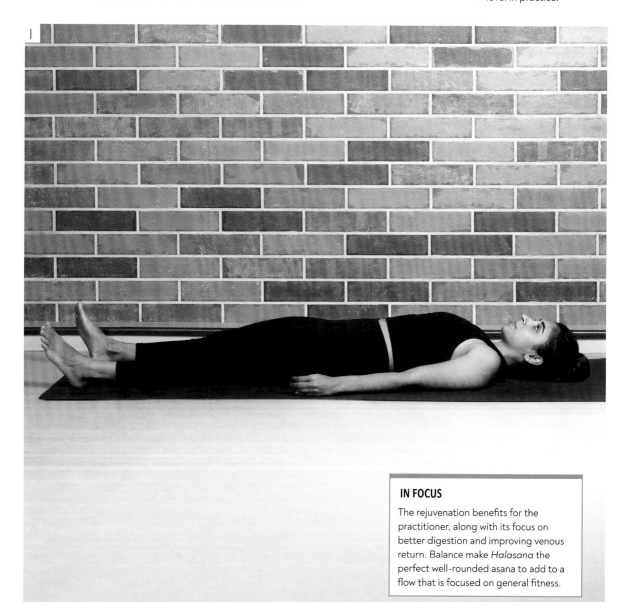

IN FOCUS

The rejuvenation benefits for the practitioner, along with its focus on better digestion and improving venous return. Balance make *Halasana* the perfect well-rounded asana to add to a flow that is focused on general fitness.

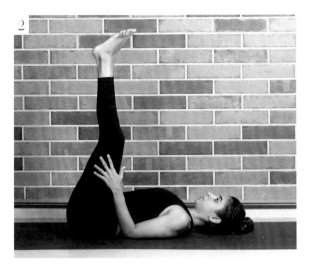

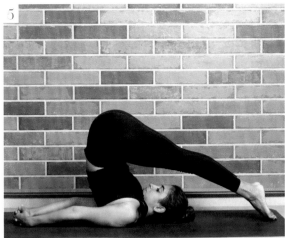

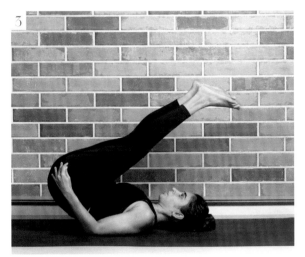

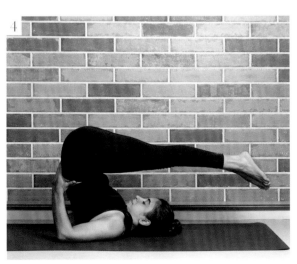

1 Lie on the back and take a few calm and deep breaths. In this position, the legs should be joined and hands on either side of the body with palms facing up.

2 Raise both legs off the ground until perpendicular by engaging the core muscles. Maintain a compact and straight stance. The hands can rest on the thighs.

3 Slowly raise the glutes and hips off the ground. Roll the spine until the feet lift up and behind the head. The legs should remain straight.

4 Keep pushing the legs backwards by raising the back. Spine should be straight and hands back on the ground. Bring the toes down as much as possible.

5 Push until the toes touch the ground. The arms should rest naturally on the ground, with fingers intertwined. Hold for five breaths or until comfortable.

ANAND BALASANA

Also called the "happy baby pose", this soothing yoga asana is ideal for beginners and great for stretching out the body completely. When in this pose, the practitioner resembles a baby joyfully lying on their back, which is what gives it the English name.

BENEFITS & CARE

The asana improves hip mobility, stretches hamstrings, strengthens arms, and calms the mind. If suffering from a back ailment, bend the knees and keep feet flat. Avoid when distracted or disturbed as it could lead to headaches or dissatisfaction. Avoid practising at the end of a pregnancy.

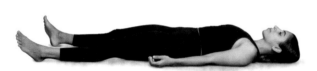

Lie flat on the back on the ground, feet slightly apart. Keep the arms relaxed on either side of the body, palms facing up.

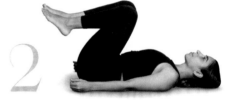

Inhale while bringing the knees to the chest at a 90-degree angle. Be sure to keep the head flat on the ground and the gaze straight upwards.

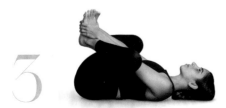

Hold the feet from the inside of the knees and gently spread the knees. The knees should be in line with the armpits and the gaze should be upwards.

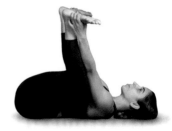

Point the soles of the feet upwards. Allow the length of the arm to touch the length of the shin. Sway from side to side for a few moments while taking deep breaths.

SUPERHUMAN | *Anand Balasana*

MATSYASANA

Matsyasana translates to the "fish pose" as *matsya* means "fish" in Sanskrit. It gets its name from the final pose which resembles the marine creature. This reclining and back-bending asana offers a full stretch of the body.

BENEFITS & CARE

Matsyasana can stimulate the pancreas, controlling blood sugar levels, tone muscles in the chest and abdomen, alleviate menstrual pain, and improve respiratory health. Avoid in case of hernia, peptic ulcers, high blood pressure, or spinal issues.

1

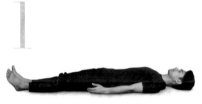

Lie in a relaxed position on the ground with the palms facing upwards.

2

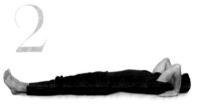

Raise arms to curl over the shoulder, pressing palms flat on the ground. Keep in position by rolling shoulders back. Expand the chest and feel the flex.

3

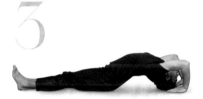

Stretch the throat by lifting the neck until the crown rolls to rest on the ground. This should create an arch of the back, lifting it away from the ground.

4

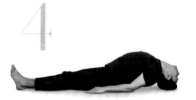

Keep the toes wiggling and move the legs at short intervals. Keep the head in position, but bring the hands back. Press the palms onto the ground.

5

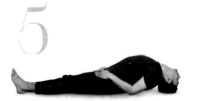

Letting the elbows remain in position touching the ground, bring the hands to rest on the thighs.

6

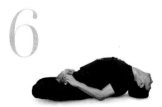

Flex and engage the forearms to press into the thighs to maintain the position of the head. Hold for a few breaths, then release the pose and return to the start.

SALABHASANA

Salabhasana is practised with a single, powerful muscle contraction, similar to a locust jumping. This asana brings together thought, breath, and movement. Practitioners do not need to lift themselves very far off the ground to gain the benefits of this pose.

BENEFITS & CARE

Salabhasana strengthens arm muscles, shoulders, abdomen, lower back, and legs. The pose also promotes a healthy digestive system, eases gastric discomfort, and reduces flatulence. Those with recent or chronic injury to the hips, knees, or shoulders should avoid it.

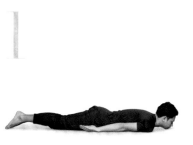

Lie on the abdomen with the legs outstretched, heels together, and toes pointed. Keep the elbows close together.

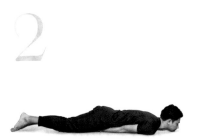

Place the chin forwards on the mat and tuck the hands flat underneath the body. Shoulders should touch on the ground.

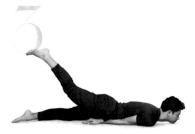

With an inhale, contract the lower back and gently raise the right leg off the ground. Ensure the knee is not bent.

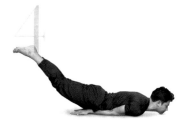

To come into the full pose, with a quick, strong inhale, contract the lower back and push on the arms. Swing both legs up as high as possible and hold the pose.

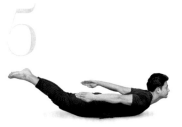

Lift the head and continue looking ahead. Bring both arms back above the hips and feel the stretch. Hold for five breaths.

IN FOCUS

Salabhasana is impactful for general fitness goals as it benefits both mind and body. Elongating the spine in this way helps to counteract poor posture and related issues, as muscles along the back and legs are engaged to hold each end of the body off the ground. Regular practise of this asana also helps one develop and strengthen the will power.

MAKARASANA

With regular practice of *Makarasana*, also known as the "crocodile pose", one can train their bodies to breathe from the abdomen, pulling focus away from the chest. This helps relieve physical and mental fatigue and calm.

BENEFITS & CARE

Makarasana is a healing posture for many types of back pain, including slipped disc, sciatica, and lower back pain. Hand and leg position can be adjusted according to practitioner's comfort. Do not attempt if pregnant, or suffering from low blood pressure or heart conditions.

1

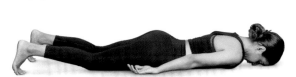

Lie flat on the stomach, feet hip-width apart, and the arms by the side. Rest the forehead and the chin on the floor. Aim to release the body's weight.

2

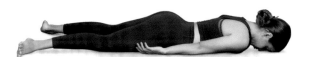

Let the feet fall to the sides and take a few deep breaths. There is nowhere to focus and the eyes and mind are resting in emptiness. Dwell on that awareness.

3

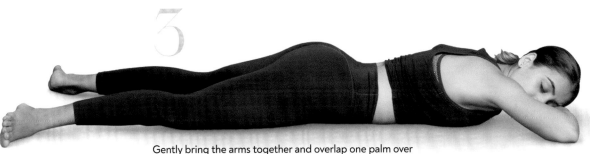

Gently bring the arms together and overlap one palm over the other. Rest the head over the hands and close both eyes. With each breath, feel the abdomen move against the floor.

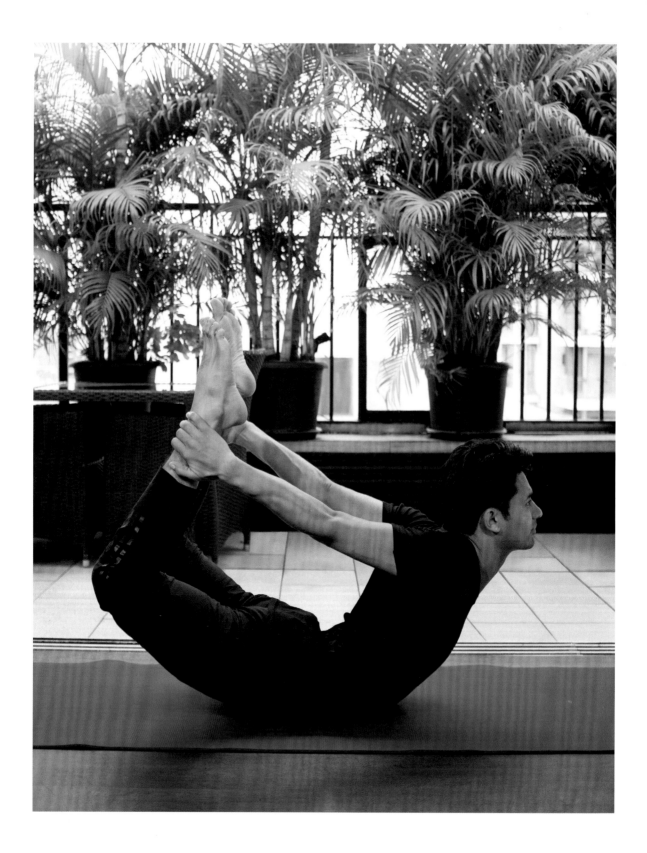

DHANURASANA

A deep opening up of the chest muscles and a full stretch are the highlights of *Dhanurasana*, which translates to "bow pose". The taut posture of the body resembles the weapon in its final pose. This asana is best approached once the practitioner has gained some experience as the balance it requires can be tricky for a beginner.

BENEFITS & CARE

Dhanurasana tones the abdominal muscles and the back, strengthens ankles, thighs, chest, neck, and shoulders, improves digestion, facilitates better breathing, and can help cure neck pain. Best to avoid this in case of neck or spinal injuries, pregnancy, migraine, irregular blood pressure, hernia, or peptic ulcers.

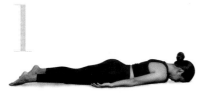

Lie in the prone position and keep both feet apart in line with the hips. Arms should rest on either side of the body.

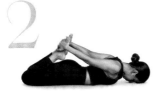

Fold the legs at the knees and grip both ankles by extending the hands backwards. Head should be straight with the crown touching the ground.

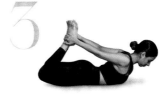

Inhale deeply and lift the chest off the ground while still looking down. Raise the legs up and backwards as well.

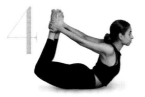

Look straight ahead and continue to lift as much of the chest and legs off the ground as is comfortable to do without pain.

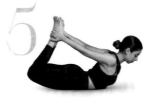

Do not overextend the body's limits. Hold briefly, then slowly relax the stance along with a deep and slow inhalation.

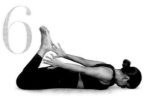

Exhale after 15–20 seconds while lowering the torso back to the ground. Relax and release the grip on both ankles when ready.

KONASANA

Also known as the "angle pose" or "sideway bending pose", *Konasana* derives its name from Sanskrit, wherein *kona* means "angle" and asana means "pose". This essential posture centres the body and mind, and it has many variations depending on the practitioner's level of comfort.

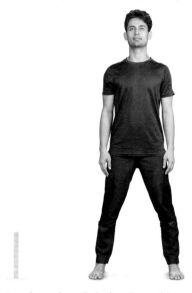

Stand upright with the legs hip-width apart. Maintain a straight spine and look ahead.

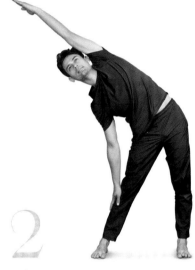

With an inhale, raise the left arm and bend sideways till the left ear touches the upper. Rest the right palm by the knee.

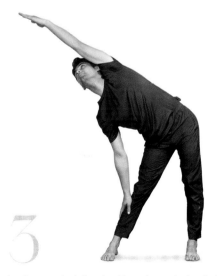

Look up at the left palm. Try to keep the heels, hips, head, and shoulder in one line. Maintain equal weight on both the legs.

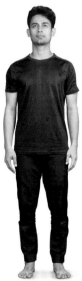

Exhale and return to upright position and drop the hands to the side. Repeat on the other side two or three times.

UPAVISTHA KONASANA

Upavistha Konasana offers intense stretch of the upper and lower body, and has a calming effects due to forward bends. This pose enhances the connection between the body and breath, lengthens the hamstring, stretches the back, and increases mental calmness.

BENEFITS & CARE

A great asana for the joints, the groin, and abdomen muscles, the *Upavistha Konasana* also enhances spinal flexibility and relieves fatigue and anxiety. Don't practise it if pregnant, or suffering from hip, back, or wrist injury.

IN FOCUS

Upavistha Konasana is included in general fitness flows for its overall impact on the body. It strengthens the muscles and helps regulate blood flow. The gentle bends prevent hernia and relieve sciatica pains. Practising this posture also helps in regularizing the menstrual flow in addition to stimulating the functioning of ovaries.

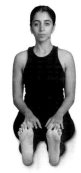

1

Sit with the back straight and legs stretched out in front. Keep the toes flexed and the knees straight. Hands should rest on the thighs and with a straight chin, look ahead.

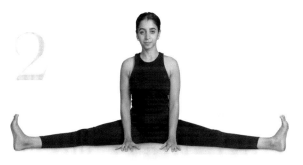

2

Spread the legs as wide as possible, while keeping the spine straight. Try to position the legs at a 90-degree angle to the pelvis, or in a straight line. Place the hands on the ground.

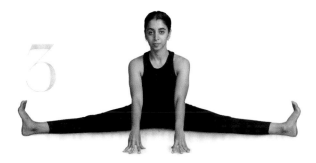

3

With a deep inhale, slowly bend the upper body forwards. Let the hands slide up ahead or crawl with the hands to lower the body as far as possible on the ground. Keep the legs stable.

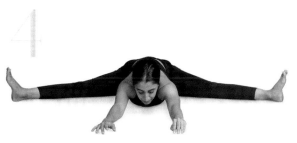

4

In the final pose, the torso should be parallel to the ground and the arms should be stretched out in front. Hold this pose for five breaths, then slowly return to the sitting position.

NATARAJASANA

An intermediate asana within yoga, the *Natarajasana* challenges the practitioner to surrender to the body and open up the hips and the heart. When done regularly, it can do wonders for one's strength and balance.

BENEFITS & CARE

Natarajasana aids in better breathing, strength, posture, and flexibility. Do not perform if suffering from weakness, any injuries or pain, or if feeling distracted or stressed.

IN FOCUS

Adding the *Natarajasana* to the general fitness flow has great benefits. It is an excellent asana to perform for building stamina and durability. It strengthens the core, back, hips, thighs, ankles, hamstrings, calves, and shins, while also improving one's balance and breathing.

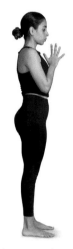

1 Stand with feet slightly apart. Take a deep breath. Join the palms and keep eyes fixed on a single object. Get ready to balance on one leg.

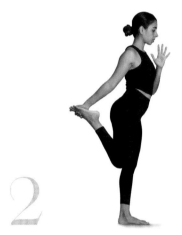

2 Bend the right leg and bring it close to the glutes and hold the foot with the right palm. Carefully free the left hand while maintaining balance. The gaze should remain fixed.

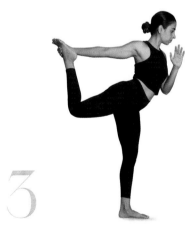

3 Concentrate all the body weight on the left leg and slowly extend the right leg as far back as possible, while bending forwards in a controlled manner.

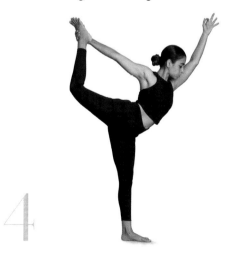

4 Raise the right leg higher, while also raising the left hand. Raise them as high as possible. Hold this pose for five breaths. Return to the starting position and repeat with the left leg.

UTTANASANA

The Sanskrit word *uttana* translates to "great stretch", which is what gives this asana its name. True to its name, *Uttanasana* opens up the muscles in the hips, hamstrings, and back, bringing the body to a state of intense stretching.

BENEFITS & CARE

Uttanasana lengthens the spine and stimulates the digestive, uro-genital, nervous, and endocrine systems. Do not perform in case of recent injuries or irregular blood pressure.

IN FOCUS

For fitness enthusiasts, not only is *Uttanasana* a wonderful way to stretch and support the musculoskeletal system, but it also reduces abdominal fat, aids balance, improves the functioning of the nervous and digestive systems, and helps with better sleep.

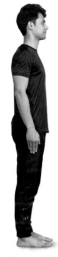

1 Start by standing straight with both feet together. Place both arms to the side of the body, and take in regular breaths.

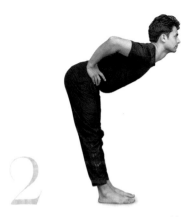

2 Bring the hands to cup the waist and begin to lean forwards. Bow the head first, then bend the lower trunk, followed by the top trunk.

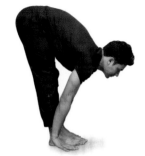

3 Place both palms down on the ground, making sure to keep the elbows and knees straight. Take a deep breath and prepare to go down lower.

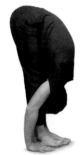

4 Try to touch the forehead to the knees and feel the bend at the hips. Back should be straight. If unable to touch the knees with the head, go as far down as possible.

VIRABHADRASANA I

The "Warrior I", or *Virabhadrasana I*, is symbolic of power, stability, and deep focus. The standing pose is beginner-friendly and stretches the front the body and is great for building strength in the legs, core, and back. Similar lunging standing poses are also performed by gymnasts and martial artists.

BENEFITS & CARE

Virabhadrasana I improves concentration and balance, relieves stiffness in the back, neck, and shoulders, and is beneficial in overcoming arthritis. Those who are pregnant, or have hip, knee, shoulder, or back injuries should avoid the pose.

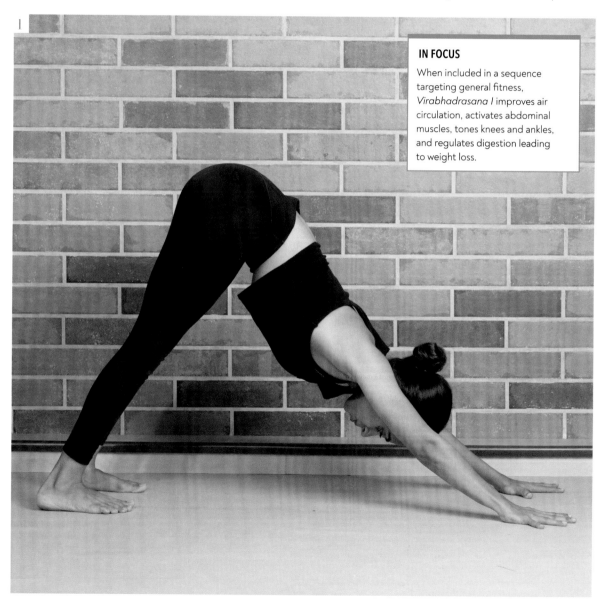

IN FOCUS

When included in a sequence targeting general fitness, *Virabhadrasana I* improves air circulation, activates abdominal muscles, tones knees and ankles, and regulates digestion leading to weight loss.

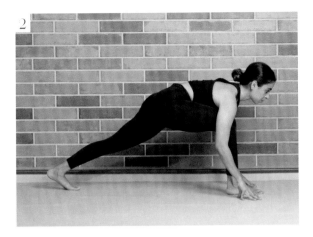

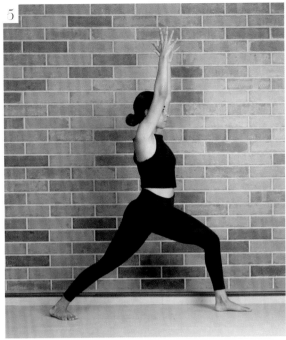

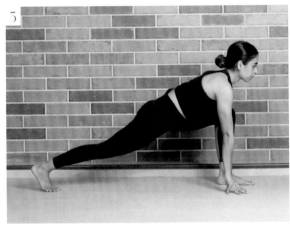

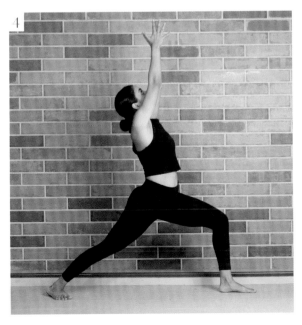

1 Start in *Adho Mukha Shvanasana* (see p52) with the hips raised and the body forming a triangle.

2 Bring the left foot forwards so that the toes are in line with the fingers. Shift the foot slightly to the left. Hips should be lowered and the head straightened.

3 Bend the left knee and stretch the right leg back till it rests on the toes. The knee should be in line with the ankle and the left outer hip should be pinned back.

4 Lift the torso up until upright, raise both arms such that palms are facing each other. Inhale and let the shoulder blades expand up and outwards, away from the spine.

5 Gaze should be set at the thumbs but can be straight ahead. Hold the pose for five breaths. Return to the starting position and repeat on the other side.

WE ARE A LITTLE PIECE OF CONTINUAL CHANGE, LOOKING AT AN INFINITE QUANTITY OF CONTINUAL CHANGE.

B.K.S. IYENGAR, FOUNDER OF IYENGAR YOGA

SAVASANA

In this asana, the practitioner assumes a supine position and allows the mind and body to completely relax. To the observing eye, this appears to be the position of a corpse – arms outstretched, slow, natural, almost invisible breaths – which gives it its name. Ideally, the deceptively simple-seeming *Savasana* lasts for at least 10 minutes, but can also be carried out for 20 minutes or more depending on the level of practice.

BENEFITS & CARE

Savasana relieves physical and mental stress from the body by easing fatigue and relaxing the limbs. Regular practice can also ease hypertension and improve sleep. Those who are pregnant, or suffer from chronic back pain or acidity should practise this under supervision, or avoid it.

1

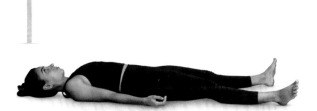

Lie down in a supine position with arms at a 15-cm distance from the body and shoulders relaxed. Palms should be turned up and fingertips curled. Close the eyes. Clear the mind, breathe deeply, and remain still. Stay in this position as long as needed.

2

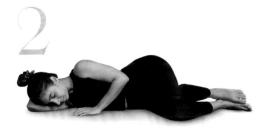

Gradually, become aware of the body, starting from the right foot, the right knee, and continuing to the hip. Repeat with the left leg and continue to think of the body up to the head. Roll to the left and stay in position with the eyes shut. Inhale and exhale slowly.

3

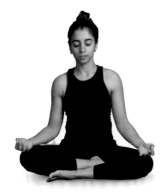

Gently sit up in a relaxed, cross-legged position, with the help of hands pressing on the ground. Once seated, keep the eyes closed and continue breathing slowly. Rub the palms together and press them to the eye lids, to warm the eyes. Open the eyes slowly.

IN FOCUS

Including the *Savasana* in one's yoga fitness journey enables the body to reset, refresh, and repair itself. At the end of a practice, with Savasana, the practitioner is able to allow the effects of the rest of the yoga sequence to permeate through the mind and body. This makes the asana important within any flow.

CHANDRA BHEDANA PRANAYAMA

Chandra Bhedana Pranayama, or "left nostril breathing", involves deep breathing, prolonged breath retention, and deep exhalation. It comprises Sanskrit words *chandra*, or the "moon", *bhedana*, meaning "piercing", and pranayama, or breathwork. This is a simple and effective breathing technique that helps cool down the body.

I

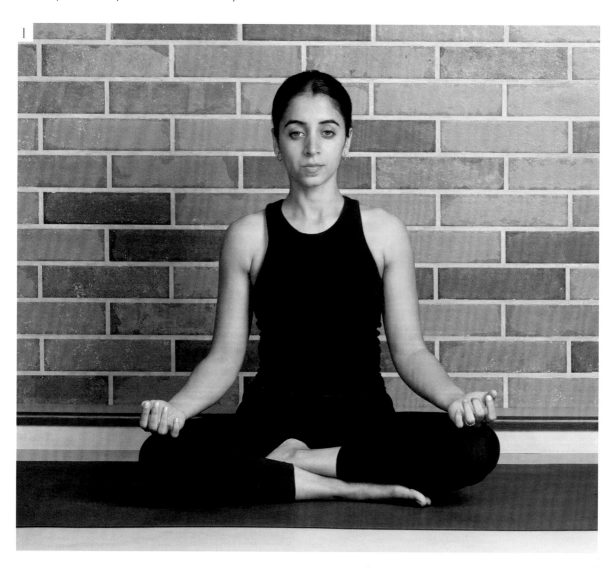

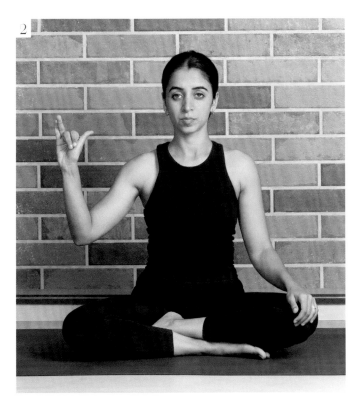

1 Choose a comfortable cross-legged position such as *Sukhasana* (see pp34–35) to sit on the ground. Keep the head straight and align it with the spine. Both hands should be on the knees with the palms facing upwards and the mind should be relaxed.

2 On the right hand, press the index and middle fingers towards the thumb. Keep both eyes open and gaze firmly ahead. Breathe regularly while preparing to do the pranayama.

3 Bring the index and thumb of the left hand together. This is the *Gyan Mudra*. Close the right nostril with the right thumb (if left-handed, then close the right nostril with the index and middle fingers of the left hand and perform the pranayama with the left hand). Inhale with the left nostril and let the air fill the lungs. Hold this breath for as long as comfortable, then slowly exhale through the right nostril. Try to exhale for longer than the inhalation.

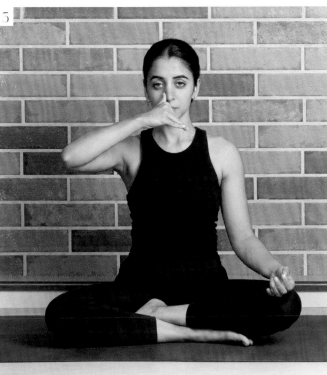

BENEFITS & CARE
This asana relieves heartburn, and refreshes and energizes the mind and body. Avoid if suffering from hypertension, heart disease, and epilepsy.

SURYA BHEDANA PRANAYAMA

Also known as "right-nostril breathing", *Surya Bhedana Pranayama* balances the nervous system and calms a hyperactive mind. This breathing technique has a host of benefits for the mind and body and, as it generates heat in the body, its practice is beneficial during winters.

BENEFITS & CARE

A deeply relaxing pose, *Surya Bhedana Pranayama* boosts energy, makes the mind more alert, and helps deal with low blood pressure. Avoid if suffering from hypertension, heart disease, and epilepsy.

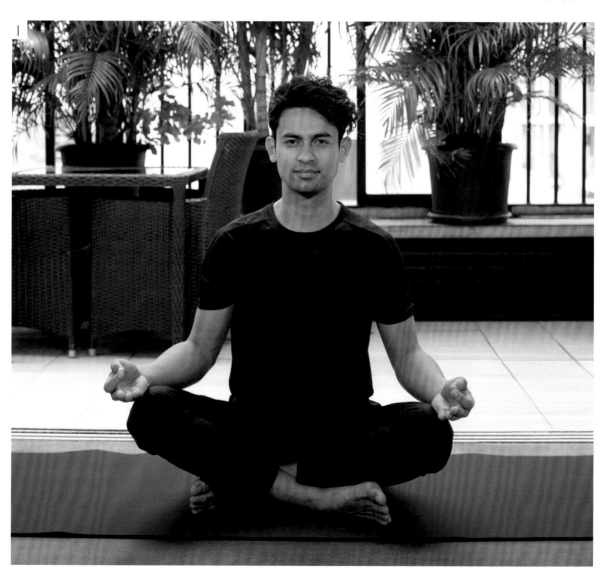

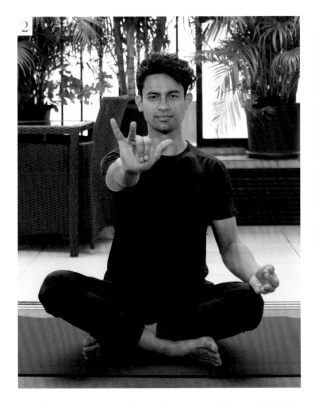

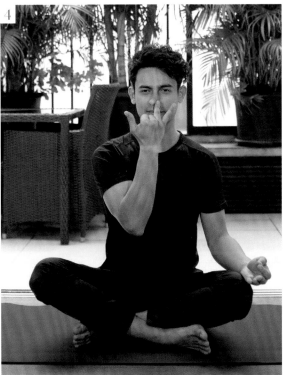

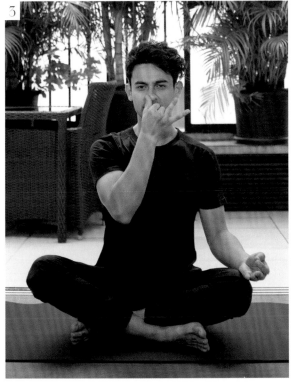

1.   Choose a comfortable cross-legged position such as *Sukhasana* (see p151) to sit on the ground. Keep the head straight and align it with the spine.

2.   With the right hand, make the *Mrigi Mudra* by pressing the index and middle fingers towards the thumb. Keep the left hand in *Gyan Mudra*, with the index finger and the thumb together.

3.   Close the left nostril with the ring finger. Take a deep breath from the right nostril and seal it shut with the right thumb. Continue to hold your breath.

4.   Lift the ring finger off the left nostril while keeping the right nostril closed with the thumb. Exhale deeply and repeat the asana for two or three minutes.

SITKARI

Aptly called "hissing breath" to denote the sipping action or hissing sound that prevails during this pranayama, or breathwork, *Sitkari* is a cooling exercise for the mouth, throat, and chest. In this, breath is drawn into the lungs through clenched teeth and exhaled after a period of hold in one long exhalation.

BENEFITS & CARE

Sitkari is good for digestive function, regulating blood pressure, maintaining body temperature, and relieving anxiety. Avoid this in case of heart ailments, migraines, or very low blood pressure.

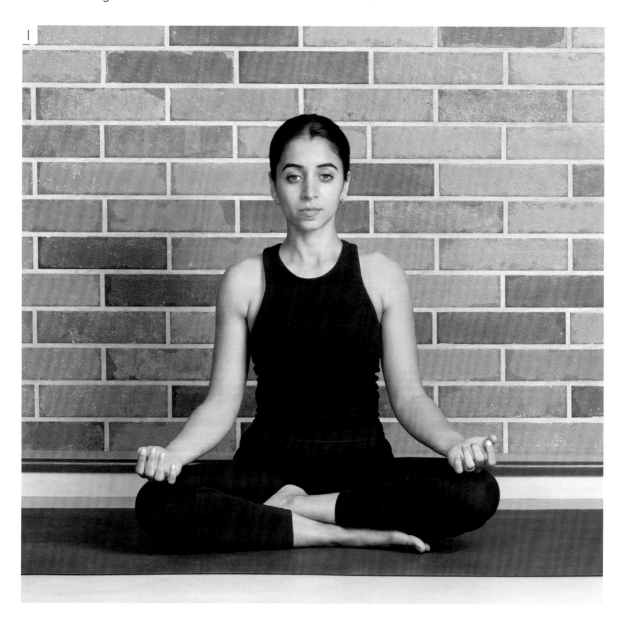

1

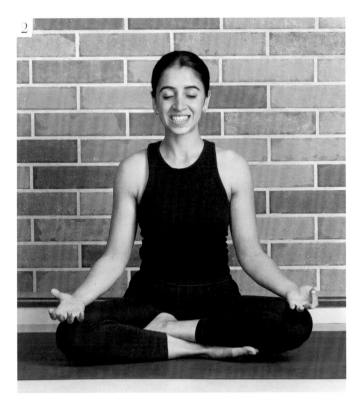

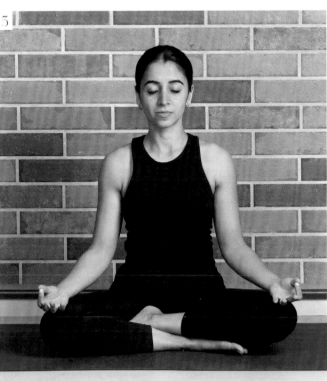

1 Assume the *Sukhasana* (see p151). Be sure to align the body in a straight line, while still being comfortable in the posture. Close both eyes and place hands on the knees. Join the tips of both index fingers to the tips of the thumb, applying light pressure. This is the *Gyan Mudra*.

2 Gently press the top and bottom teeth together so that they are exposed to the air. The lips should be set comfortably apart to facilitate this. The bottom of the tongue should contact the upper palate when curled upwards. If unable to curl the tongue, simply rest it behind the teeth. Inhale slowly and deeply through the spaces between the teeth. A small hissing sound will be heard on inhalation. Feel the air fill the chest and neck first, then the abdomen.

3 After a few moments, seal the lips, then seal the entire mouth area, such that the act of breathing naturally shifts to the nose on the exhale. The breath going out should be calm and controlled. This is the first round of the *Sitkari* pranayama. Repeat as many times as comfortable.

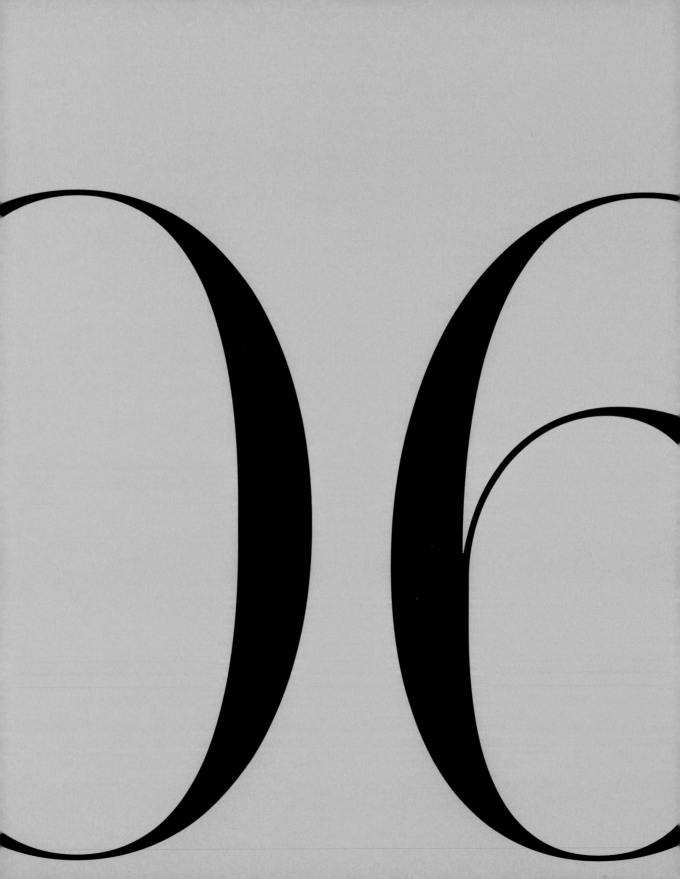

SURYA **NAMASKAR**

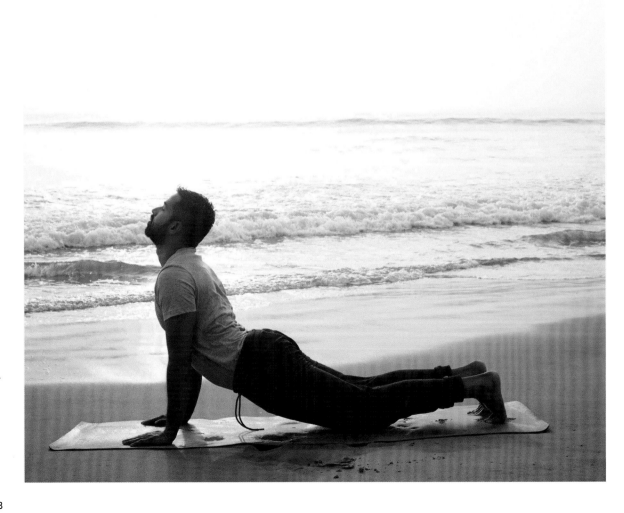

SALUTATIONS TO
THE SUN

The *Surya Namaskar*, or sun salutations, as they are popularly called, is perhaps one of the most dynamic yoga sequences in the practice. Dedicated to the Hindu sun god, Surya, the sequence started out as flowing movement-based prayers, performed even today in parts of India, at sunrise or sunset.

T. Krishnamacharya, the guru of modern Yoga, has been credited with the sequence's addition to yoga in the 20th century. Today, it has become an essential part of the practice – its importance evident in its many benefits.

With its sequence of 12 steps, the versatile *Surya Namaskar* is a great warm-up, when practised before any activity, sport, or a trip to the gym. It helps one get a good, and sometimes, much-needed stretch, opening up the entire body from head to toe. It improves blood circulation

and strengthens the bones and muscles. The focus on inhaling and exhaling makes it an excellent training for breathwork.

The sequence can also be incorporated into a yoga flow or practised on its own. The asanas making up the sequence can be modified, removed, or variations introduced to suit the practitioner's needs or fitness levels. It is why anyone, no matter what their age, can perform the *Surya Namaskar*.

This is especially true of *Surya Namaskar B* (see pp182–185), which is a perfect standalone sequence. In fact, a combination of the *Surya Namaskar* and *Anulom Vilom* (see p109) is a good way to begin one's journey into yoga. Start with performing the *Surya Namaskar* six times (three on each side), ending with breathwork, slowly increasing the number over time.

SURYA NAMASKAR A

The "sun salutations", or the *Surya Namaskar*, are a series of different asanas practised in succession. Although there are several variations, this one is ideal for a beginner and is great as a simple warm-up flow that readies the body for more elaborate practice.

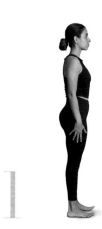

1 Begin by placing both feet hip-width apart and standing with feet firmly planted on the mat or ground. Arms should be relaxed on either side and head facing straight in front.

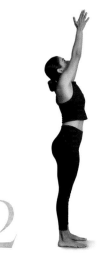

2 Join both palms together, with space between the thumbs and fingers. On an inhalation, sweep the arms upwards and turn to the sky. The back should be gently arched.

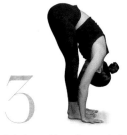

3 Exhale and lean forwards, bending at the hips. Reach for the ground with both hands, palms open and touching the mat. Bring the nose to the knees, bending them if needed.

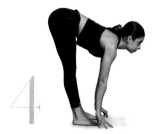

4 Take a deep breath and raise the body, stretching the spine. The back should be straight and parallel to the ground. Touch the ground with the fingertips.

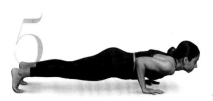

5 Breathe out and take a step back, then go down into a plank pose. It should resemble a high push-up with feet apart and hands tucked under the shoulders.

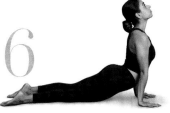

6 Bring the legs to the mat and arch the chest up. Straighten both arms and pull back with the shoulders, almost as though raising the heart to the sky.

> "
> You have got all the materials inside for
> wisdom, for becoming a Yogi or *Jnani* [wise].
> Practise. Develop. Assert. Realize.
>
> SWAMI SIVANANDA SARASWATI, NOTED YOGA GURU AND PHYSICIAN
> "

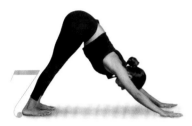

7. Slowly plant the feet on the ground. Exhale and raise the hips while bringing the chest down to resemble a mountain. Hold for five breaths, then bend the knees and turn the head between both arms

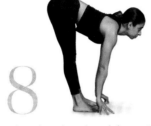

8. Take a deep breath and then stride to bring both feet forwards, by the hands. Raise the chest up to straighten the back and bring it parallel to the mat again. Bring the tips of the fingers to rest on the ground.

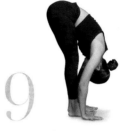

9. Exhale and slowly lower the upper body down to touch the thighs and bring the nose to the knees. Hands can be on the ground by the feet, or on the shins, as comfortable.

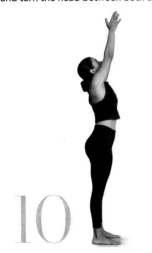

10. Breathing in deeply, raise the body to an upright position with the arms stretched upwards and the palms joined together. Look up to the sky with a gently arched back

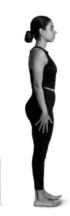

11. Let out the breath and lower the arms down to either side of the body, returning to the starting position. Prepare to run through the sequence again.

BENEFITS & CARE

Surya Namaskar A can be used as a complete exercise routine. It stretches muscles in the arms and legs, tones the abdomen, relieves constipation, and leads to weight loss. Avoid in case of weakness, back pain, or weak ankles or wrists.

SURYA NAMASKAR B

This is a slightly advanced version of the *Surya Namaskar* with 19 steps and the inclusion of more complicated asanas, such as *Virabhadrasana I* (see pp92–93). This sun salutation has a vast and positive impact on mental and physical health.

BENEFITS & CARE

Surya Namaskar B activates the quadriceps, works the cardiovascular system, and functions as a great standalone fitness exercise. Do not perform in case of shoulder injury, a weak heart, or in case of a fever.

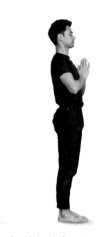

1 Stand with both feet together. Bring the hands together, palms facing each other in a prayer position. Place the thumbs on the sternum and inhale deeply.

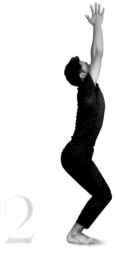

2 Inhale and bend the knees. Arch the back gently and assume a chair-like position, pushing the hips down. Raise the arms up straight and keep the hands joined and fingers splayed.

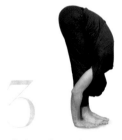

3 Exhale and straighten the legs, then bend at the hips and fold the body forwards. Bring the nose to the knees and place the hands on the ground by the feet. Bend the knees if needed.

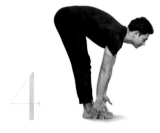

4 While raising the body up, take a deep breath in. Bring the fingertips to the shins or keep them on the ground.

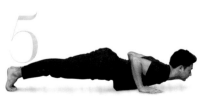

5 Breathe out and step or jump back. Lower the body to the ground into a plank-like pose. Body weight should be on the toes and palms of the hand.

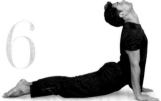

6 Rest the legs on the mat and arch the chest up. Straighten both arms and pull back with the shoulders, almost as though raising the heart to the sky.

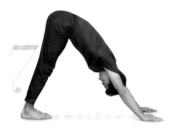

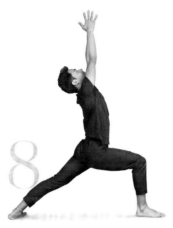

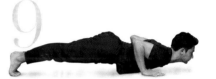

Slowly plant the feet on the ground. Exhale and raise the hips while bringing the chest down to resemble a mountain. Stretch the spine and push the belly and hips upwards.

Inhale and with the left heel on the ground, slide the right foot forwards. The right knee should bend, but the rear leg should remain straight. Lift the arms into the air and look up.

Slowly bringing both feet back together, lower the body, and return to the position in step 5. Exhale and hold the pose for a few moments.

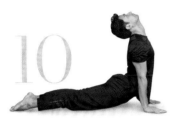

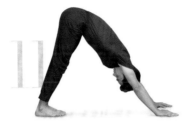

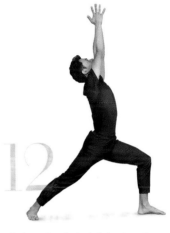

Rest the legs on the mat and arch the chest up to resemble the pose in step 6. Straighten both arms and pull back with the shoulders.

Slowly plant the feet on the ground. Exhale and raise the hips to match the position in step 7. Stretch the spine and push the belly and hips upwards.

Inhale and with the left heel on the ground, slide the right foot forwards to resemble step 8. Lift the arms into the air and look up.

> **"**
> Inhale, and God approaches you.
> Hold the inhalation, and God remains with
> you. Exhale, and you approach God. Hold
> the exhalation, and surrender to God.
>
> T. KRISHNAMACHARYA, AUTHOR AND YOGA TEACHER
> **"**

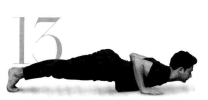

13 Slowly bringing both feet back together, lower the body, and return to the position in step 5. Exhale and hold the pose for a few moments.

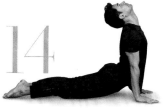

14 Rest the legs on the mat and arch the chest up to resemble the pose in step 6. Straighten both arms and pull back with the shoulders.

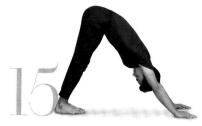

15 Slowly plant the feet on the ground. Exhale and raise the hips to match the position in step 7. Stretch the spine and push the belly and hips upwards.

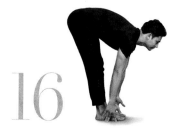

16 Take a deep breath and step or jump forwards, bringing both feet together by the hands. Stretch the spine and keep the back parallel to the ground. Bring the fingertips to the shins or keep them on the ground.

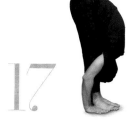

17 Exhale and straighten the legs to match step 3, then bend at the hips and fold the body forwards. Bring the nose to the knees and place the hands on the ground by the feet. Bend the knees if needed.

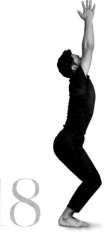

18 Inhale and bend the knees to match step 2. Arch the back gently and assume a chair-like position, pushing the hips down. Raise the arms up straight overhead and keep the hands joined and fingers splayed.

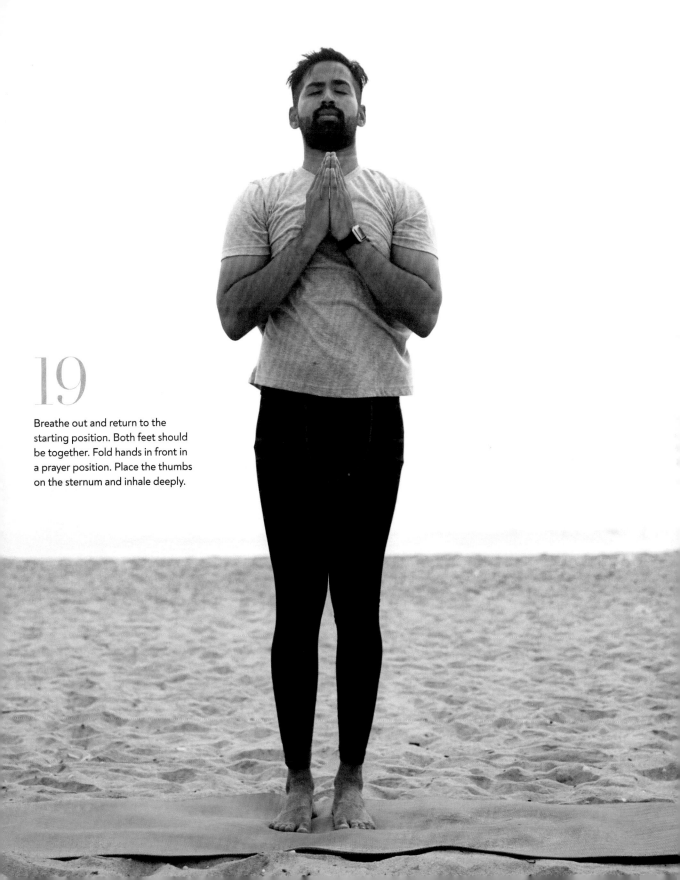

19

Breathe out and return to the starting position. Both feet should be together. Fold hands in front in a prayer position. Place the thumbs on the sternum and inhale deeply.

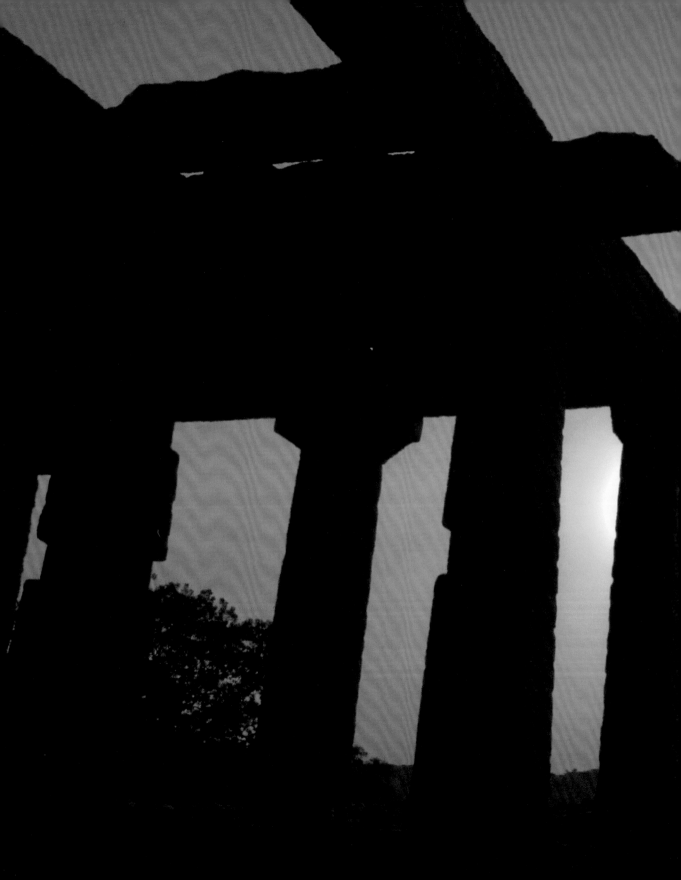

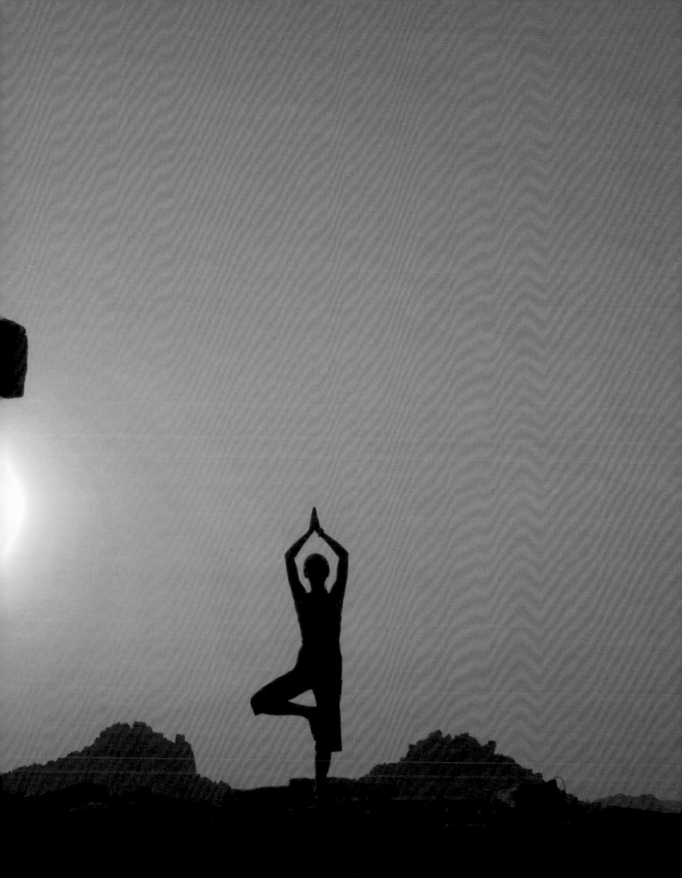

INDEX

ACKNOWLEDGMENTS

ABOUT THE AUTHOR:
Sarvesh Shashi is the brain behind Diva Yoga, a consumer health platform built on the authentic foundations of yoga to solve six primary health goals. Having seen the benefits of yoga and mindfulness firsthand since the age of 6, Sarvesh wanted to help others in their quest for a healthier lifestyle. At 21, he set up a studio chain that flourished over the next years across India, with a vision to connect seven billion breaths. He built upon this and is today the founder and head coach at Diva Yoga. His aim is to make yoga-based wellness a part of the modern lifestyle, to combat global epidemics like stress, anxiety, depression, sleeplessness, and obesity. He is also a travel and adventure enthusiast and has played cricket professionally for about 17 years.

AUTHOR'S ACKNOWLEDGMENTS:
Malaika Arora, co-founder of Diva Yoga and actor, for her support and encouragement, and for sharing images.

Janhavi Saraf and Dhiral Sampath for content curation, and Abhilash Gowda and Basavaraj Saunshi for providing content for "In Focus" boxes.

PUBLISHER'S ACKNOWLEDGMENTS:
Beat Dance Studio, Santacruz, and Beat Dance Studio, Khar, for providing studio space, Vinay Kumar for all model photography, and Devashish Dhoundiyal, Shraddha Iyer, and Jahnavi Patwardhan for modelling.

Nayan Keshan for editorial support and assistance, Vatsal Verma for proofreading, Bhavika Mathur for design support, and Manpreet Kaur for picture research administration support.

Disclaimer:
Every effort has been made to acknowledge those individuals, organizations, and corporations that have helped with this book and to trace copyright holders.

DK apologizes in advance if any omission has occurred. If an omission does come to light, DK will be pleased to insert the appropriate acknowledgment in the subsequent editions of the book.

The publisher would also like to thank the following for their kind permission to reproduce their photographs:

(Key: a-above; b-below/bottom; c-centre; f-far; l-left; r-right; t-top)

4 Nithin Bharath. 7 Nithin Bharath. 8 Avinash Gowariker. 12 Nithin Bharath. 14 Nithin Bharath. 16 Nithin Bharath. 18 Nithin Bharath: (tl, br). Dreamstime.com: Fizkes (tr). Unsplash: (bl). 21 P Thaniesthaban. 22-23 Nithin Bharath. 26 Nithin Bharath. 29 Nithin Bharath. 31 Nithin Bharath. 34 Nithin Bharath. 38 Riddhi Parekh. 44-45 Getty Images / iStock: E+ / aluxum. 46 Nithin Bharath. 50-51 Dreamstime.com: Svyatoslav Lypynskyy. 59 Riddhi Parekh. 62 Nithin Bharath. 64-65 Alamy Stock Photo: Glenn Ruthven. 76 Amar Ramesh. 78-79 Amar Ramesh. 80 Nithin Bharath. 88-89 Alamy Stock Photo: David Jennings. 96 Dreamstime.com: Nipa Sawangsri (Background). Avinash Gowariker: (cb). 112 Getty Images: Moment / Elizabeth Fernandez. 115 Dreamstime.com: Yuri Arcurs (t); Vadym Pastukh (b). 123 P Thaniesthaban. 127 Avinash Gowariker: (c). Unsplash: NordWood Themes (Background). 136-137 Dreamstime.com: Fizkes. 142 Nithin Bharath. 145 Nithin Bharath. 147 Nithin Bharath. 152 P Thaniesthaban. 178 Nithin Bharath. 185 Nithin Bharath. 186-187 Getty Images: RooM / inigoarza

All other images © Dorling Kindersley Limited

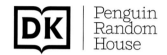

DK DELHI
Project Editor Avanika
Senior Art Editor Devika Awasthi
Jacket Designer Neha Ahuja Chowdhry
Managing Editor Chitra Subramanyam
Managing Art Editor Neha Ahuja Chowdhry
DTP Designers Umesh Singh Rawat, Rajdeep Singh
DTP Coordinator Tarun Sharma
Pre-Production Manager Balwant Singh
Production Manager Pankaj Sharma
Managing Director, India Aparna Sharma

DK LONDON
Art Director Maxine Pedliham
Editorial Director Cara Armstrong
Publishing Director Katie Cowan

Photographer Vinay Arora
Jacket Designer Eleanor Ridsdale

First published in Great Britain in 2024 by
Dorling Kindersley Limited
DK, One Embassy Gardens, 8 Viaduct Gardens,
London, SW11 7BW

The authorised representative in the EEA is
Dorling Kindersley Verlag GmbH. Arnulfstr. 124,
80636 Munich, Germany

A CIP catalogue record for this book is available
from the British Library.
ISBN: 978-0-2416-3341-0

Printed and bound in India

www.dk.com

This book was made with Forest
Stewardship Council™ certified
paper – one small step in DK's
commitment to a sustainable future.
Learn more at
www.dk.com/uk/information/sustainability